First Choice Cookbook

Fast & Easy
Low Fat, Low Sugar Recipes

By Colleen Bartley

Picnics Publishing
Sechelt, B.C., Canada

First Choice
Cookbook

By Colleen Bartley

First Printing
Copyright © Colleen Bartley 2001

Canadian Cataloguing in Publication Data

Bartley, Colleen, 1953-
First Choice Cookbook

Includes Index.
ISBN 0-9680037-3-7

1.Diabetes--Diet therapy--Recipes. 2. Low-fat diet--Recipes 3. Sugar-free diet--Recipes.
RC662.B368 2001   641.5'6314   C2001-910869-9

Published by Picnics Publishing
P.O. Box 2461, Sechelt
British Columbia, Canada
V0N 3A0
Fax: (604) 885-4375

Printed & bound in Canada by Friesens Printers

Table of Contents

Author's Acknowledgements

Writing a cookbook is a huge undertaking, which requires many different skills and areas of expertise. I am very grateful to the many friends, family, and co-workers who so enthusiastically offered their unique talents, time, energy, and hard work in order to produce the *First Choice Cookbook*.

First and foremost I would to thank Doreen Yasui, the dietitian at B.C.'s Children's Hospital. Doreen has been my mentor for two books. She has cheerfully spent hours and hours ensuring that the information is relevant and correct and that this book is a useful tool for people with diabetes.

I would also like to thank Alison Evert for her careful review, her helpful suggestions and for embracing this project with such positive enthusiasm.

To the artist Tara Reed, goes my appreciation for taking my ideas and making them better that I could imagine with her vision and artistry.

I am thankful that I know many 'computer experts' that were willing to help. Nathan Koss, Clive Lloyd, Heather Bartley, Kevin Doyle, and Geoff Reed, were all instrumental in design and production.

Finally, thanks to all of the other friends and family who spent time tasting, testing, typing, editing, and fine-tuning the recipes and for all of their love and support.

Colleen Bartley

Dedication

This book is dedicated to the memory of Rob Hagen.
I was lucky to know this very special man for a short while and I will always be grateful for his encouragement and his belief in me.

Foreword

The *First Choice Cookbook* is full of delicious recipes that are quick and easy to prepare. This cookbook is perfect for a busy family or the cook that wants to prepare healthy foods without having to spend hours in the kitchen. Colleen Bartley has included many practical 'how to tips' that make this cookbook a great investment.

She has also calculated the exchange values for each of the recipes that she has created for the *First Choice Cookbook.* However these recipes are not just for people with diabetes; they can be enjoyed by everyone in the family.

I hope that you enjoy making these healthy and fun recipes!

Alison B. Evert, RD, CDE
Registered Dietitian and Certified Diabetes Educator

Introduction

When first diagnosed with diabetes one can suddenly feel overwhelmed by a new world of dietary restrictions. Whether a small child or an adult, being faced with the prospect of no longer being able to eat what you like is at once daunting and depressing.

When writing the 'Kid's Choice Cookbook' I tried to determine what kids liked (based on my family and friend's tastes) and then developed and adapted recipes that were satisfying but low in fat and sugar. The reaction that the 'Kid's Choice Cookbook' received convinced me that the book was both timely and appreciated. The basic recipes and the emphasis on cooking for fun appealed to many families. Also, the easy instructions and familiar ingredients made anyone struggling with a new way of cooking less intimidated.

With this in mind I went to work on the 'First Choice Cookbook'. I used the foods and recipes that my family liked as a starting point for this book as well. I decided to call it the 'First Choice Cookbook' because of the simple recipes for all 'first time' cooks and for people learning to cook a 'low fat', 'low sugar' diet.

All of the recipes are kitchen tested by my family and friends. They include easy-to-follow instructions, helpful hints, and are enjoyable to make and to eat. I have employed a variety of basic cooking skills as well as methods to change traditionally fatty recipes into lower-fat alternatives. I hope that the techniques and hints help new cooks to adapt their own favorite recipes.

Food and cooking should always be one of life's pleasures. Diet and exercise continue to be the best way to control blood sugar levels, but your new 'meal plan' doesn't have to be a sentence to a lifetime of sensible, boring meals. Approach this new diet with a sense of adventure. Try the new 'low-sugar, low-fat' choices appearing on the grocery store shelves. Try all the new fruits, vegetables, herbs, and ethnic foods now available. Your meal plan can be and should be a delicious, fun-filled challenge that results in better eating for everybody!

"Cooking is like falling in love; it should be done with abandon or not at all."

Important tips to know when using this book:

☺   The recipes in this book use the Exchange Values of the American Diabetes Association. The book is intended for use with the advice of a dietitian and following a meal plan devised by your dietitian.

☺   Calculations were done using the 'Food Quest Program', which is based on the Canadian Nutrient File. In the case of new products not in the program, information from manufacturers and on manufacturers' labels was used.

☺   Unless otherwise stated, all recipes in this book were tested and analysed using 1% milk, 0.1% yogurt, 5% sour cream, 1% cottage cheese, partly skimmed (less than 20% M.F.) Mozzarella & Cheddar cheeses, water packed tuna, and juice packed canned fruits. Some 'no-fat' ingredients such as sour cream are suggested toppings but not successful ingredients when cooked.

☺   In some recipes optional toppings are suggested. These are not used in the calculations of the Exchanges. If you are not sure how optional foods will affect the Exchange Value per serving, ask your dietitian.

☺   The grams of carbohydrate in the Food Choice Values of some recipes may seem lower than the grams of carbohydrate stated in the recipe. This is because the grams of fiber have been subtracted from the total carbohydrates before the Exchange Values were calculated.

☺   Meat exchanges usually have some fat included but proteins from legumes and grains do not have the fat found in a meat-based Meat Exchange. Therefore, the fat contained in a Meatless Main Dish is assigned a Fat Exchange.

☺   Now that foods containing sugar can be eaten in moderation by people with diabetes, some prefer it to sugar substitutes. Your dietitian can explain how to include sugar in your diet.

Meal planning approaches

A meal plan is not a diet, but a guide to assist people with diabetes in choosing healthy meals and snacks. The meal plan can help you to keep your blood glucose levels in desirable ranges. A registered dietitian can help design an individualized meal plan that fits your unique lifestyle. When creating a meal plan for you, the registered dietitian will consider a number of following factors:

* Age
* Lifestyle - what is your work or school schedule?
* Activity
* Medication - diabetes medicine as well as other types of medicine
* Weight goals
* Usual eating habits and food preferences
* Other medication conditions
* Blood glucose monitoring records

The registered dietitian will also provide you with some nutrition education about how the different foods you eat can effect your blood glucose level. A meal plan can help you coordinate your food intake with the action of the insulin or diabetes medication in your body. Food is made up of three main fuels: carbohydrate, protein, and fat.

Blood Glucose Response To The Three Main Fuel Sources:

Carbohydrate
* Most important aspect of the meal plan.
* Carbohydrate foods include starches and bread, fruit, and milk.
* Main source of blood glucose. Approximately 90-100% of dietary carbohydrate enters the blood stream as glucose within 15 minutes to 1-2 hours.
* Greatest determinant of amount of insulin needed to control the blood glucose level after meals.
* Consistency in amounts eaten at meal and snacks makes it easier to fine tune diabetes medications.

Protein

*   Approximately 50-60% of the dietary protein is converted to glucose and released into the bloodstream. This process occurs 2 to 5 hours following meal/snack.
*   Protein foods include meat, fish, poultry, eggs, cheese, peanut butter, and meat alternatives.
*   Protein adds "staying power" to your meals and snacks.

Fat

*   Negligible (less than 10%) effect on the blood glucose level.
*   Delays/slows the digestive process.
*   Heart healthy foods are recommended for people with diabetes as they have a greater incidence of heart disease.
*   Consumption of fat may need to be monitored more closely in situations of co-existing obesity.

Two commonly used meal planning approaches for people with diabetes are Exchange Lists or Carbohydrate Counting.

Exchange Lists

Commonly eaten foods are grouped into six different exchange groups. The Exchange Lists groups include the following:

*   Starch
*   Fruit
*   Milk
*   Vegetable
*   Meat/Protein foods
*   Fat

Each exchange within a group is an amount of food with a set nutritional value. Therefore, foods in each specific Exchange List can be substituted or "exchanged" with other foods from the same list. The Exchange List approach allows for a meal plan guide to be consistent while offering a wide variety of food choices. An individual with diabetes using this approach has a prescribed number of exchanges to be consumed at meal and snack times. Substitutions between exchange groups containing carbohydrate can be made to increase flexibility. For example: 1 Starch exchange can be substituted for 1 Fruit exchange or 1 Milk exchange.

The author of the *First Choice Cookbook* has calculated the exchange values of all of the recipes.

Carbohydrate Counting

This approach emphasizes the carbohydrate content of the food. The registered dietitian teaches the person with diabetes how to determine the carbohydrate content and/or the grams of carbohydrate in foods consumed at meals and snacks. This information is obtained from the Exchange Lists and from the nutrition information on food labels. Carbohydrate Counting provides increased flexibility in meal planning while keeping the amount of carbohydrate consistent from day to day. Foods in the meat and fat groups contain little carbohydrate and therefore are not used in this approach.

1 carbohydrate choice = 1 Starch Exchange = 15 grams of Carbohydrate
1 Fruit Exchange
1 Milk Exchange

And finally a word about sugar. Sugar is okay, sugar is not a poison! Small or calculated amounts of sugar are acceptable in a diabetes meal plan. Research does not support the long held theory that ingestion of sugar can dramatically increase your blood glucose level. Foods containing sugar can be substituted for part of the carbohydrate foods allowed in your meal plan. It is recommended that these "empty calorie" foods do not replace healthy foods on a regular basis. You will find a few recipes in the *First Choice Cookbook* that include small amounts of sugar. The sugar content of these recipes have been included into the total carbohydrate content of the recipes and are reflected in the exchanges listed at the bottom of each recipe.

TIPS FOR HEALTHY EATING TO ACHIEVE OPTIMAL BLOOD GLUCOSE CONTROL

* Try to eat meals and snacks at regular times everyday.
* Be consistent: eat about the same amount of food at meals and snacks each day.
* Sugar does fit occasionally into a diabetes meal plan when substituted for other carbohydrate foods.
* Eating healthy foods and meals takes a little extra time and planning, but the rewards are great. Try to plan a few meals each week, using resources like the *First Choice Cookbook* will make this task much easier!
* Low blood glucose (hypoglycemia) can occur in the absence of regular meals and snacks if you take diabetes medications to help you control your blood glucose levels. Be sure to check with your physician or registered dietitian to see how your diabetes medication can effect your blood glucose level.

Painless ways to "slim" your recipes:

☑ Substitute low fat or non-fat sour cream for regular. Evaporated milk (2% or skim) can replace cream in most recipes. There is a great new product available in the U.S. by Land-o-Lakes called "Fat-free Half & Half"

☑ For gratin toppings that are made of crumbs & butter, reduce the amount of butter and then spray the top of the casserole with cooking spray. This will result in a nicely browned surface without as much fat.

☑ Switch to low fat cream soups in recipes calling for canned soups, such as Campbell's 98% Fat Free® or Healthy Recipe®.

☑ Use non-stick fry pans and minimal oil or butter for sautéing or stir-frying

☑ Instead of sautéing vegetables in butter for casseroles etc.; wash, place in microwave-safe dish, cover with plastic wrap and steam until tender crisp, then add to recipe.

☑ Buy strongly flavored versions of high fat ingredients, e.g. Sharp cheese or extra virgin olive oil, a smaller amount gives lots of flavor.

☑ Substituting some of the fat with applesauce or fruit purees in baking provides moistness and flavor. However you will need to consider the increased amount of carbohydrate that the applesauce contributes to the recipe.

☑ Cocoa powder is lower in fat than chocolate squares, with just as much flavor.

☑ Try substituting low-fat turkey sausage for pork sausages in your recipes. One ounce of turkey sausage contains about 57 calories and 4 grams of fat compared to pork sausage at 96 calories and 8 grams of fat.

The Best Way To:

Hard cook eggs - Place eggs in a pot with enough water to cover. Bring water to a boil. Cover pot and remove from heat. Let stand for 15 minutes. Cool eggs under cold running water.

Cook corn on the cob - Remove husks and silks. Add corn to a large pot of boiling salted water. Return to a boil and cook four minutes only.

Bake a potato - Scrub a russet potato and prick several times. Bake at 425°F for 55-60 minutes.

Seed an avocado - Cut lengthways & rotate both halves to separate. Insert knife firmly in pit, twist and lift out.

Cook white rice - Bring rice, 1 tsp. salt and double the amount of water to a boil. Reduce heat, cover tightly and simmer 20 minutes or until the water is absorbed. For brown rice, cook 45 minutes.

Separate an egg - Crack open a cold egg. Holding each half pour back and forth between the halves letting the white drip into a bowl.

Clean mushrooms - Wipe with a damp paper towel. Rinse quickly with water if very dirty.

Ripen peaches, nectarines, plums, pears, or tomatoes - Place in a plain paper bag and close top. Do not refrigerate.

Chop an onion - Cut a peeled onion in half from stem to root end. Lay onion half flat on cutting board. Make horizontal cuts, then vertical cuts almost to the root end. Slice across cuts.

Hull strawberries - Just before using, rinse and then remove caps with a light twist or using the point of a sharp paring knife.

Appetizers & Snacks

Cajun Chicken Fingers

8 halves (2lbs)	Chicken breasts, boneless, skinless
3 tbsp	Paprika
2 tbsp	Brown sugar
1 tsp	Cumin, ground
1 tsp	Cayenne pepper
1 tsp	Allspice
1 tsp	Salt
1/2 tsp	Garlic powder

1. Preheat broiler. Lightly coat broiler pan with cooking spray. Cut each chicken breast into 4 long strips.
2. Mix remaining ingredients in a medium sized mixing bowl. Add chicken strips and toss, evenly coating with spice mixture
3. Place chicken strips on prepared pan in a single layer. Broil, turning once, for 6-8 minutes or until no longer pink in the center.
4. Garnish with lemon wedges and serve with 'Dude Ranch Dip'.

Dude Ranch Dip:

In a food processor (or small bowl) combine:

1/2 cup cottage cheese	1 clove garlic, minced
1/4 cup plain yogurt	1/4 tsp pepper
2 tsp cider vinegar	2 tbsp chives, dried

Makes 16 servings.
Exchanges for each serving of
2 fingers & dip:
1/2 Vegetable
2 Very lean meat

Dude Ranch Dip
Each serving of 2 tbsp:
1/2 Lean meat
(2g carbohydrate, 4g protein, 27cal)

3g Carbohydrate, 16g Protein, 1g Fat, 92 cal
(3g available Carbohydrates)

Pastrami & Apple Snacks

24 slices	Cocktail rye bread
1/4 cup	'Light' mayonnaise
1 tbsp	Prepared horseradish
1/3 lb	Deli style turkey pastrami
2	Red apples, cored
1 cup	'Light' Swiss cheese, grated

1. Preheat oven to 450°F.
2. Place rye slices in a single layer on an ungreased baking sheet.
3. Combine mayonnaise and horseradish in a small bowl. Spread on top of rye slices. Divide pastrami evenly on top of horseradish spread. Core apples and cut each one into 12 thin slices. Top pastrami with an apple slice and then the grated cheese.
4. Bake for 3 - 4 minutes, just until the cheese melts.

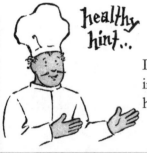

healthy hint...

Luncheon meats and prepared cold cuts are often high in fats. At the deli choose turkey breast, roast beef, ham, pastrami or corned beef as 'lean' alternatives.

Makes 12 servings.
Exchanges for each serving of 2 slices:
1/2 Starch
1 Medium-fat meat

11g Carbohydrate, 8g Protein, 4g Fat, 117 cal
(11g available Carbohydrates)

Mexican Chicken Spirals

8 oz	Cooked chicken breast, finely diced
8 oz	'Light' cream cheese
1 cup	Monterey Jack cheese, grated
1/4 cup	Cilantro, chopped
2 tbsp	Jalapeno peppers, minced
1 tsp	Chili powder
1 tsp	Cumin, ground
1/4 tsp	Salt
6	8" Whole wheat tortillas

1. In a mixing bowl combine chicken, cream cheese, Monterey Jack, cilantro, jalapeno peppers and spices.
2. Spread mixture evenly over tortillas, roll each tortilla tightly. Wrap in plastic wrap and refrigerate for 2 hours or up to 24 hours.
3. Preheat oven to 350°F and spray a baking sheet with cooking spray.
4. Cut each tortilla roll into 10 slices. Arrange slices in a single layer on prepared baking sheet, spray tops with cooking spray.
5. Bake for 12-15 minutes or until lightly browned. Serve hot with salsa.

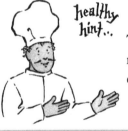

healthy hint...

There are many great fresh and bottled salsas at the market. They are usually low in fat & sugar and an easy way to add interest and flavor to your cooking.

Makes 20 servings.
Exchanges for each serving of 3 slices:
1/2 Starch   1/2 Fat
1 Lean meat

6g Carbohydrate, 8g Protein, 5g Fat, 101 cal
(6g available Carbohydrates)

Stuffed Mushroom Caps

32	Large Mushrooms
6 oz	'Light' cream cheese
1/2 cup	'Light' Swiss cheese, grated
4 oz	Crab, fresh or canned
2 tbsp	Chives, snipped
1 clove	Garlic, minced

1. Preheat oven to 375°F. Clean and remove stems from mushrooms. Place caps upside down on a paper towel and microwave for 2 minutes, until slightly softened.
2. Place right side up on a baking sheet & pat dry with a paper towel.
3. In a small mixing bowl combine remaining ingredients, spoon into caps.
4. Bake for 10 to 12 minutes, until hot and cheese is melted. Serve hot.

chef's secret...

Soaking canned crab in cold water before using freshens the flavor. Soak for 10 minutes, drain well and then pat dry with paper towels.

Makes 8 servings.
Exchanges for each serving of 4 mushrooms:
1 Vegetable
1 Medium-fat meat

5g Carbohydrate, 10g Protein, 6g Fat, 107 cal
(5g available Carbohydrates)

Thai Kabobs

4- 4oz	Chicken breasts, boneless, skinless
1/4 cup	'Light' mayonnaise
1/3 cup	Fat-reduced peanut butter
1/3 cup	Chicken broth
3 tbsp	Soy sauce
2 tbsp	Splenda®
1 tsp	Garlic powder
1/2 tsp	Ginger, ground
1/4 tsp	Tabasco sauce

1. Cut each chicken breast lengthwise and at an angle into 8 strips. Put into a plastic bag.
2. Combine remaining ingredients in a small mixing bowl. Save half of the sauce for dipping and add the other half into the plastic bag with the chicken strips, coating strips evenly. Press out the air and seal the bag.
3. Marinate in the refrigerator 8 hours, turning the bag occasionally.
4. Soak 32 wooden skewers in water for 30 minutes. Thread chicken strips accordion-style onto skewers. Discard marinade.
5. Broil (or grill) about 4 minutes per side until slightly browned and cooked through. Serve with reserved sauce for dipping.

Makes 16 servings.
Exchanges for each serving of 2 kabobs:
1/2 Vegetable
1 Lean meat

3g Carbohydrate, 8g Protein, 3g Fat, 70 cal
(3g available Carbohydrates)

Pizza Potato Skins

3/4 lb (6 small)	Russet potatoes
1	Green or red pepper, diced
1/2 cup	Onions, diced
2 cloves	Garlic, minced
4 oz	Turkey salami, chopped
1 cup	Marinara sauce
1 tsp	Oregano, dried
1 cup	Part skim Mozzarella cheese, grated

1. Bake potatoes at 400°F for 50 - 60 minutes, until soft. Allow to cool. Decrease oven temperature to 350°F.
2. Lightly coat a non-stick frypan with cooking spray. Add peppers, onions, and garlic. Cook over medium high heat for 3 - 4 minutes or until softened. Stir in Marinara sauce, chopped salami, and oregano. Set aside.
3. When potatoes are cool enough to handle; cut in half & scoop out potato pulp leaving a 1/2" shell. Cut shells in half lengthwise again. Place on an ungreased baking sheet.
4. Spoon sauce mixture onto shells. Sprinkle with grated Mozzarella.
5. Bake at 350°F for 15 to 20 minutes, until cheese is melted.

time for
a change

Vary this recipe by using leftover chicken, turkey, or ham instead of the turkey salami.

Makes 8 servings.
Exchanges for each serving of 3 skins:
1 Starch
1 Medium-fat meat

23g Carbohydrate, 9g Protein, 6g Fat, 190 cal
(23g available Carbohydrates)

Pepper Cheese Squares

1/2 cup	All purpose flour
1 tsp	Baking powder
1/2 tsp	Salt
8	Large eggs
1 1/2 cups	'Light' Cheddar cheese, grated
1 cup	'Light' Monterey Jack cheese, grated
1 1/2 cups	Cottage cheese (1%)
2 tbsp	Jalapeno peppers, diced
1	Red pepper, diced
12 large	Black olives, sliced

1. Preheat oven to 350°F. Lightly coat a 9" x 13" baking dish with cooking spray.
2. Stir together flour, baking powder, & salt.
3. In a separate mixing bowl beat eggs with an electric mixer on high. Stir flour mixture into eggs, mix until well combined. Fold in grated cheeses, cottage cheese, peppers, & olives.
4. Pour into prepared baking dish and bake for 40 minutes, until set. Remove from oven and let cool slightly.
5. Cut into 36 squares and serve warm.

.

Makes 36 servings.
Exchanges for each serving of 1 square:
1/2 Vegetable
1/2 Lean meat

2g Carbohydrate, 5g Protein, 2g Fat, 81 cal
(2g available Carbohydrates)

Bruschetta Turnovers

2 cups	Tomatoes, chopped
1/4 cup	Green onions, chopped
2 tbsp	Fresh Basil, (or 1 1/2 tsp dried)
1/2 tsp	Garlic powder
1/2 tsp	Pepper
1 1/2 cups	Part Skim Mozzarella cheese, grated
4	8" Whole wheat tortillas

1. In a medium sized bowl combine chopped tomatoes, green onions, snipped basil, garlic powder, & pepper.
2. Sprinkle 1/4 of the cheese over half of each tortilla. Top with tomato mixture. Fold each tortilla in half over filling.
3. Spray tops lightly with cooking spray.
4. Broil under preheated broiler (or spray bottoms & grill over medium coals for 4 -5 minutes). Turn carefully, spray lightly with cooking spray and continue cooking for 4 -5 minutes, until tortillas are golden and cheese is melted.
5. Cut each turnover in half to make two wedges.

To use fresh basil; remove stems, rinse & dry the leaves, chop or snip with scissors. Use four times as much as you would dried. Basil wilts & bruises easily so it only lasts about three days.

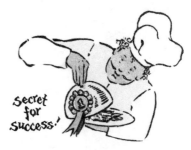

Secret for Success!

Makes 4 servings.
Exchanges for each serving of 2 wedges:
1 Starch   2 Medium-fat meat
1/2 Fruit

24g Carbohydrate, 17g protein, 11g fat, 252cal
(24g available Carbohydrates)

Mushroom Pizza Bread

1 1/2 cup	All purpose flour
1 1/2 tsp	Baking powder
1/2 tsp	Salt
3/4 cup	Light beer
1/2 cup	Spaghetti sauce
1 cup	Mushrooms, sliced
1/2 cup	Edam cheese, grated

1. Preheat oven to 425°F. Lightly coat a 9" square baking pan with cooking spray.
2. Combine flour, baking powder, & salt in a medium sized mixing bowl. Add beer and stir with a fork until blended.
3. Spread dough in prepared pan. Spread tomato sauce over the dough. Sprinkle with mushrooms and top with grated cheese.
4. Bake 15 to 20 minutes or until toothpick inserted in the center comes out clean. Cut into 16 squares and serve warm.

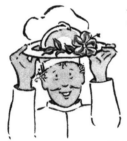

Make it Special!

Vary this recipe by using exotic mushrooms and your own favorite cheese; and/or try substituting pesto sauce for tomato sauce.

Makes 8 servings.
Exchanges for each serving of 2 squares:
1 Starch   1/2 Fat
1 Vegetable

**22g Carbohydrate, 5g Protein, 3g Fat, 143 cal
(22g available Carbohydrates)**

Tortilla Pizza Melts

1	can (14oz)Black beans
1/2 tsp	Garlic powder
2 tsp	Chili powder
4	8" Whole wheat tortillas
3	Tomatoes, thinly sliced
2 tbsp	Jalapeno peppers, chopped
1 cup	Part skim Mozzarella cheese, grated
2 tbsp	Cilantro, snipped

1. Drain and rinse beans. Mash lightly with a fork. Stir in garlic powder & chili powder.
2. Spread on tortillas, dividing evenly among them. Sprinkle each with 1/4 cup cheese. Top with tomato slices and jalapeno peppers. Sprinkle with remaining cheese and garnish with cilantro.
3. Bake at 400°F for 5 to 7 minutes, until tortilla edges are brown & crisp and the cheese is melted.

time for a change

For a great addition to a Tex-Mex BBQ these tortillas can also be cooked on the grill: Barbeque 3-4 minutes, until the cheese melts, then cut into wedges and serve as an appetizer.

Make 4 servings.
Exchanges for each serving of 1 tortilla melt:
3 Starch
1 1/2 Medium-fat meat

45g Carbohydrate, 19g Protein, 11g Fat, 337 cal
(45g available Carbohydrates)

Marinated Shrimp

1/2 lb	Cooked Shrimp, fresh or frozen
2 tbsp	Olive oil
2 tbsp	Parmesan cheese, grated
2 cloves	Garlic, minced
1/2 tsp	Pepper
1/4 tsp	Salt
2 tbsp	Lemon juice
32 slices	Cocktail rye bread

1. Coarsely chop shrimp (thaw first if frozen). Combine with remaining ingredients, except cocktail rye, in a small mixing bowl.
2. Marinate for at least an hour in the refrigerator.
3. Serve on cocktail rye. Garnish with parsley or dill sprigs and little lemon wedges.

time for a change

For an easy 'make ahead' appetizer stuff marinated shrimp into lettuce-lined mini pita pockets and garnish with fresh dill.

Makes 8 servings.
Exchanges for each serving of 4 shrimp-topped rye slices:
1 Starch
1 Lean meat

14g Carbohydrate, 9g Protein, 4g Fat, 129 cal
(14g available Carbohydrates)

Spinach Dip

1 cup	Onions, chopped
2 clove	Garlic, minced
1	pkg (10oz) frozen Spinach, thawed & squeezed dry
2/3 cup	'Light' sour cream
1/2 cup	'Light' mayonnaise
1 tbsp	Vinegar
1 tsp	Salt
1 tsp	Dill weed, dried
1/4 tsp	Cayenne pepper
1 1/2 cups	Water chestnuts, chopped

1. Put chopped onions and garlic in a microwave safe bowl, cover with plastic wrap and micro-cook for 2-3 minutes, until onions are softened. Let cool. Transfer to a food processor (or mixing bowl).
2. Add other ingredients, except water chestnuts. Process (or stir) until chunky. Add water chestnuts and stir just until mixed.

Make it Special!

Serve in a sourdough bread bowl: cut off the top of a 6" round loaf leaving a 1 1/2" border, scoop out dough. Spoon dip into shell and surround with vegetable dippers. If you eat the bread bowl don't forget to count it as a starch serving!

Makes 12 servings.
Exchanges for each serving of 1/3cup:
1/2 Starch
1/2 Fat
Does not include exchanges for vegetable dippers

6g Carbohydrate, 1g Protein, 3g Fat, 68 cal
(6g available Carbohydrates)

Layered Mexican Dip

1	can (14oz) fat-free Refried beans
1/2 cup	Salsa
1 1/2	Avocados
2 tsp	Lemon juice
6	Green onions, chopped
1/4 cup	'Light' mayonnaise
1 clove	Garlic, minced
1 1/2 cups	'Light' sour cream
1 cup	'Light' Cheddar cheese, grated
1/4 cup	Black olives, sliced
2	Tomatoes, chopped

1. Refried bean layer: In a small mixing bowl, combine the refried beans and the salsa. Spread in a 9-10" pie plate.
2. Process avacado & lemon juice in food processor, until smooth. Add garlic, 1/2 green onions & mayonnaise, process again. Spread over refried beans.
3. Dollop sour cream onto guacamole layer and carefully spread to cover all.
4. Sprinkle cheddar cheese, tomatoes, remaining green onions, & olives on top in concentric circles or diagonal stripes. Serve with tortilla chips for dipping.

Make it Special!

For Hallowe'en cover the dip with grated cheese & then use the toppings to make a Jack'O'Lantern face. For Christmas make the dip in a Christmas tree pan with the toppings arranged like garlands.

Makes 15 servings.
Exchanges for each serving of 1/4cup:

1/2 Starch	1/2 Lean meat
1/2 Vegetable	1 Fat

  Does not include exchanges for tortilla chips

10g Carbohydrate, 5g Protein, 7g Fat, 131 cal
(10g available Carbohydrates)

Salads & Sides

Greek Romaine Salad

3 tbsp	Feta cheese, crumbled
3 tbsp	Red wine vinegar
2 tbsp	Olive oil
1 clove	Garlic, minced
1/2 tsp	Oregano
1/2 tsp	Pepper
1 large head	Romaine lettuce
1 cup	Zucchini, julienned
1/2 cup	Red onions, thinly sliced
1	Pepper, red or green, diced
16	Cherry tomatoes, halved
1/4 cup	Black olives, sliced
1/4 cup	Feta cheese, crumbled

1. To make the dressing: process the first 6 ingredients in a food processor (or blender) until smooth.
2. Tear romaine into bite size pieces. Toss with zucchini, onion, pepper, and cherry tomatoes in a large salad bowl. Drizzle with dressing & toss to mix.
3. Mound onto individual salad plates. Garnish with sliced olives and remaining feta. Serve immediately.

chef's secret...

To 'julienne vegetables' means to cut in match-stick size strips.

Makes 8 servings.
Exchanges for each serving of 1/8th recipe:
1 Vegetable   1 Fat
1/2 Very lean meat

5g Carbohydrate, 3g Protein, 6g Fat, 89 cal
(5g available Carbohydrates)

Layered Tuna Salad

4 cups	Iceburg lettuce, bite size pieces
4 stalks	Celery, sliced
2 cups	Cucumber, sliced
1/2 cup	Frozen peas, thawed
2	cans (6oz) Tuna, drained
2	Red or green peppers, diced
1/2 cup	Red onions, sliced
2 cups	Alfalfa sprouts
1/2 cup	Plain yogurt, low fat
1/3 cup	'Light' mayonnaise
1 cup	'Light' Cheddar cheese, grated
2	Tomatoes, cut in wedges
10 sprigs	Parsley

1. In a large clear bowl layer lettuce, celery, cucumber, peas, tuna, green pepper, onion and alfalfa sprouts, in order listed.
2. Stir mayonnaise and yogurt together and spread over top, completely covering salad. Sprinkle with grated cheese.
3. Cover and refrigerate 8 hours or overnight.
4. Garnish with tomato wedges and parsley sprigs.
5. Toss just before before serving.

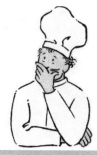

time for a change

Vary this recipe by using diced cooked chicken instead of tuna.

Makes 8 servings.
Exchanges for each serving of 1/8th recipe:
2 Vegetable
1 1/2 Medium-fat meat

**10g Carbohydrate, 16g Protein, 6g Fat, 165cal
(10g available Carbohydrates)**

New Wave Waldorf Salad

1/4 cup	Walnuts, toasted
1 bunch (10oz)	Spinach
1/4 cup	Raspberry vinegar
2 tbsp	'Light' mayonnaise
1 tbsp	Lime juice
2	Red apples, thinly sliced
2 stalks	Celery, thinly sliced
1	Yellow pepper, thinly sliced
4	Green onions, chopped
2 tbsp	Parsley, snipped

1. Chop walnuts and then toast by spreading on a baking sheet and baking at 350°F until golden and fragrant, about 5 minutes. Let cool.
2. Rinse spinach leaves well. Pat dry with paper towels and discard any tough stems. Arrange on salad plates.
3. Combine raspberry vinegar, mayonnaise, & lime juice in a small bowl.
4. Toss remaining ingredients together with vinegar mixture in a mixing bowl. Divide onto spinach. Sprinkle with toasted walnuts & parsley and serve.

chef's secret... To toast nuts without heating the oven: place them in a non-stick frypan over medium-low heat and warm them, shaking the pan occasionally, until fragrant & golden.

Makes 6 servings.
Exchanges for each serving of 1/6th recipe:
2 Vegetable
1 Fat

9g Carbohydrate, 3g Protein, 4g Fat, 85cal
(9g available Carbohydrates)

New Potato Salad

1 lb	Small new potatoes
6	Green onions, chopped
1	Red or green pepper, diced
2 stalks	Celery, thinly sliced
1/4 cup	Carrots, shredded
1/4 cup	'Light' sour cream
1/4 cup	Plain yogurt, low fat
2 tsp	Dijon mustard
1/2 tsp	Salt
1/2 tsp	Black pepper
1/2 tsp	Dill weed, dried

1. Scrub potatoes and place in a medium sized saucepan, add water just to cover and sprinkle with salt. Bring to a boil, reduce heat and simmer for 20 - 25 mins, until tender. Drain; let cool. Cut into quarters (1/2" - 3/4" pieces).
2. In a large mixing bowl combine cooled potatoes with green onions, pepper, celery, & carrots.
3. In a small bowl stir together the sour cream, yogurt, Dijon mustard, salt, pepper, & dill. Drizzle onto the potato mixture and toss gently to coat.
4. Cover and chill for 4 hours or overnight.

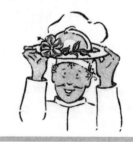

Make it Special

Make this salad colorful and appealing by using a combination of peppers; red, yellow, & green. Also, serve it in a lettuce lined bowl.

Makes 6 servings.
Exchanges for each serving of 1/6th recipe:
1 Starch

16g Carbohydrate, 3g Protein, 1g Fat, 89 cal
(16g available Carbohydrates)

Full of Beans Salad

2 cups	Fresh green beans, cut in 1" pieces
1 1/2 cups	Lima beans, frozen
1	can (14oz) Kidney beans
1	can (14oz) Garbanzo beans
1	can (14 oz) Corn
4 stalks	Celery, sliced
1	Red or green pepper, diced
1/2 cup	Red onion, chopped
2 tbsp	Olive oil
3 tbsp	Red wine vinegar
2 tbsp	Splenda®
2 cloves	Garlic, minced
1/4 cup	Parsley, snipped
1/2 tsp	Salt
1/4 tsp	Pepper

1. Bring a large pot of water to a boil. Add green beans, and frozen lima beans. Return to boil, reduce heat and simmer for 2-3 minutes until just tender-crisp. Drain and immediately plunge beans into very cold water to stop the cooking and retain the color. Drain well.
2. In a colander drain and rinse kidney beans, garbanzo beans & corn. Toss cooked beans with canned beans, corn, celery, pepper & onion in a large bowl.
3. Whisk together oil, vinegar, Splenda®, garlic, parsley, salt, & pepper. Drizzle onto bean mixture and toss gently.
4. Cover and refrigerate overnight.

Makes 8 servings.
Exchanges for each serving of 1/8th recipe:

1 1/2 Starch	1/2 Very lean meat
1/2 Fruit	1/2 Fat

35g Carbohydrate, 10g Protein, 4g Fat, 222 cal
(35g available Carbohydrates)

Curried Chicken Salad

3/4 lb	Cooked Chicken breast, diced
1 cup	Pineapple tidbits (juice pack)
1/2 cup	Celery, sliced
2 cups	Cauliflower, small florets
6	Green onions, chopped
1/4 cup	Peanuts, dry-roasted
1/4 cup	'Light' mayonnaise
1 tbsp	Lemon juice
1 tsp	Curry powder
1/4 tsp	Salt

1. Combine first six ingredients in a large bowl.
2. Combine mayonnaise, lemon juice, curry powder & salt in a small bowl.
3. Toss dressing with chicken mixture, stirring gently until mixed evenly.
4. Serve on lettuce leaves or in a lettuce lined salad bowl.

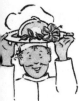

Make it Special

Curry Powder is a blend of spices that you can make yourself! In a heavy frypan over medium heat, roast 1/2 cup coriander seeds, 2 Tbsp cumin seeds, 2 Tbsp black peppercorns, 1 Tbsp sesame seeds, 1 Tbsp cardamon, & 1 or 2 dried chilli peppers. Cook 3 minutes shaking the frypan frequently, until toasted and fragrant. Transfer to a food processor and grind to a powder. Add 3 Tbsp turmeric & 2 Tbsp ground ginger: mix well.

Beware! The flavor is very intense.

Makes 6 servings.
Exchanges for each serving of 1/6th recipe:
2 Vegetable
2 Lean meat

10g Carbohydrate, 20g Protein, 7g Fat, 199 cal
(10g available Carbohydrates)

Grilled Chicken Caesar Salad

2 slices	Italian or French bread, cut in cubes
1 tsp	Garlic Powder
1 tsp	Oregano, dried
1 tbsp	Parsley, dried
2/3 cup	'Light' mayonnaise
2 tbsp	Lemon juice
2 cloves	Garlic, minced
1 tbsp	Dijon mustard
1 tsp	Worcestershire sauce
1/2 tsp	Pepper
1 1/4 lbs	Chicken breasts, skinless, boneless
2 small heads	Romaine lettuce
1/2 cup	Red onion, sliced in rings
1/2 cup	Parmesan cheese, grated

1. To make croutons: Preheat oven to 350F°. Spray a baking sheet with olive-oil flavoured cooking spray. Spread bread cubes on baking sheet and lightly coat with cooking spray. Sprinkle with garlic powder, oregano, and parsley. Bake 8-10 minutes stirring occasionally.

2. To make dressing: whisk together the mayonnaise, lemon juice, garlic, mustard, worcestershire sauce, and pepper.

3. Coat the chicken breasts with 1/4 cup of the dressing. Grill or broil 6-7 mins per side, until juices run clear when pierced with a fork.

4. Tear romaine into bite size pieces and toss with remaining dressing, onions, & croutons. Mound on plates. Slice hot chicken and fan attractively on top of romaine. Sprinkle each serving with 1 Tbsp parmesan cheese.

Makes 8 servings.
Exchanges for each serving of 1/8th recipe:
2 Vegetable
2 1/2 Lean meat

10g Carbohydrate, 22g Protein, 8g Fat, 207 cal
(10g available Carbohydrates)

Greek Tomato Bake

4	Tomatoes
1/4 cup	Red onions, diced
1/3 cup	Black olives, sliced
1/4 cup	Feta cheese, crumbled
2 tsp	Olive oil
2 tbsp	Red wine vinegar
1/2 tsp	Basil, dried
1/2 tsp	Oregano, dried
1/2 tsp	Garlic powder

1. Cut tops off tomatoes. Remove centers with a small spoon leaving a shell, invert to drain.
2. Remove seeds from tomato centers and chop remaining pulp. Mix with onions, and olives. Place tomatoes right side up in a glass dish. Spoon onion mixture back into tomato shells, sprinkle with feta. Cover and refrigerate for up to 24 hours.
3. Preheat oven to 400°F. Whisk together olive oil, vinegar, & spices.
4. Drizzle each tomato with dressing. Bake, uncovered, for 15 minutes.

Make it Special

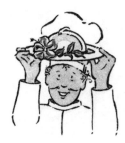

These tomatoes can also be cooked on the barbecue. They make a great side dish for shish kebabs or barbecued lamb.

Makes 4 servings.
Exchanges for each serving of 1 tomato:
1/2 Fruit   1 Fat
1/2 Lean meat

7g Carbohydrate, 3g Protein, 7g Fat, 101 cal
(7g available Carbohydrates)

Zucchini & Tomato Gratin

1 lb	Zucchini (2 small)
4	Tomatoes
1 tbsp	Fresh basil, snipped
1/2 tsp	Salt
1/2 tsp	Pepper
1/4 cup	Parmesan cheese, grated
1/4 cup	Part skim Mozzarella cheese, grated

1. Slice zucchini and tomatoes into 1/4" thick slices. Lightly coat a 9 x 13" casserole dish with cooking spray.
2. Overlap diagonal rows of zucchini and tomato slices alternately in prepared dish. Sprinkle with basil, salt, & pepper. Combine cheeses and sprinkle on top.
3. Broil 6" from heat for 5 - 6 min or until hot and cheese is lightly browned.

chef's secret...

Broiling requires very hot direct heat. Leaving the oven door open slightly when broiling allows steam to escape and ensures real broiling instead of roasting.

Makes 6 servings.
Exchanges for each serving of 1/6th recipe:
1/2 Fruit
1/2 Medium-fat meat

7g Carbohydrate, 4g Protein, 2g Fat, 62 cal
(7g available Carbohydrates)

Summer Vegetable Stir Fry

2 tsp	Olive oil
1/2 lb	Asparagus
1 cup	Mushrooms
6	Green onions, cut in 1" pces
1/2	Red pepper, thinly sliced
1 clove	Garlic, minced
1 cup	Broccoli, cut in florets
1 cup	Zucchini, diced
2 tsp	Fresh oregano, snipped
2 tsp	Fresh basil, snipped
12	Cherry tomatoes, halved
2 tsp	Soy sauce

1. Prepare vegetables: break tough stems off of asparagus stalks and discard, cut spears into 2" pieces, cut mushrooms in half or quarters if large. Prepare other vegetables as directed above.
2. Heat a large frypan or wok over high heat and add olive oil. Heat until hot but not smoking. Add mushrooms, green onions, peppers, and garlic, and stir fry for 3 mins. Add asparagus, broccoli, and zucchini. Stir fry for 2 minutes. Sprinkle with 2 Tbsp water.
3. Stir in oregano, basil, cherry tomatoes, & soy sauce. Cover and let steam for 2-3 minutes, until vegetables are tender-crisp.

Use any of your favorite fresh vegetables but cut them into even-sized pieces. Also, keep the food moving when stir-frying, if the vegetables have a chance to rest they'll steam and lose crispness.

secret for success

Makes 4 servings.
Exchanges for each serving of 1/4th recipe:
2 Vegetable
1/2 Fat

10g Carbohydrate, 5g Protein, 3g Fat, 81 cal
(10g available Carbohydrates)

Hot German Potato Salad

2 1/4lb	Small red-skin potatoes
3 slices	Pork bacon, raw
6	Green onions, chopped
1 1/2 tbsp	Grainy Dijon mustard
1 tbsp	Cider vinegar
1 tsp	Olive oil
1 tsp	Dill weed, dried
1/2 tsp	Salt
1/2 tsp	Pepper

1. Scrub potatoes and place in a large pot. Add just enough water to cover the potatoes. Sprinkle with salt and bring to a boil over high heat. Reduce heat to low and simmer for 25 minutes or until tender. Drain and set aside to cool. When cool enough to handle cut into 1" cubes.
2. Dice bacon & cook in a large non-stick frypan over medium heat until crispy Add green onions & potatoes, toss to coat with bacon drippings.
3. Stir the remaining ingredients together, drizzle over the potato mixture and toss gently. Heat over medium heat stirring occasionally for 3-4 minutes, or until heated through.
4. Transfer to a serving dish and serve hot.

Makes 6 servings.
Exchanges for each serving of 1/6th recipe:
2 Starch
1/2 Fat

29g Carbohydrate, 5g Protein, 7g Fat, 201cal
(29g available Carbohydrates)

Greek Potatoes

5 medium	Potatoes (Idaho or russet)
1 tbsp	Olive oil
1 clove	Garlic, minced
1 tsp	Rosemary, dried
1 tbsp	Lemon juice
1/2 tsp	Pepper
1/2 tsp	Salt
1/4 cup	Feta cheese, crumbled

1. Preheat oven to 425°F. Peel potatoes and cut into thick wedges. Set aside in a bowl of cold salted water to stop them from browning.
2. Heat olive oil in a small saucepan, add minced garlic and rosemary. Cook until garlic is softened but not brown. Stir in lemon juice & spices.
3. Drain potatoes and drizzle with olive oil mixture, toss lightly. Transfer to a 9 x 13" baking pan. Roast for 40-50 minutes, stirring once.
4. Sprinkle with feta cheese and serve.

time for a change

Try Mexican Potato Wedges!
Peel & cut potatoes as above. Toss with 1 Tbsp olive oil, 1/2 tsp tabasco, 1 tsp salt, 2 Tbsp chopped green onion, & 1 tsp chili powder. Top with 1/4 cup Monterey Jack cheese.

Makes 4 servings.
Exchanges for each serving of 1/4th recipe:
2 Starch
1 Fat

32g Carbohydrate, 6g Protein, 7g Fat, 207 cal
(32g available Carbohydrates)

Spicy Two Fries

1 lb (4 medium)	Baking potatoes
1/2 lb (2 medium)	Sweet potatoes (or yams)
1 tsp	Salt
1/2 tsp	Onion powder
1/2 tsp	Garlic powder
1/2 tsp	Paprika
4 tsp	Olive oil
2 tsp	Spicy Dijon mustard

1. Preheat oven to 450°F. Coat a baking sheet with cooking spray.
2. Peel and then cut potatoes & sweet potatoes lengthwise into 1/2" thick wedges. Set aside in separate bowls of cold salted water and allow to soak for 10-15 minutes. Drain and pat dry with paper towels.
3. In a small bowl combine the remaining ingredients. Spread the baking potato wedges in a single layer on the prepared baking sheet. Drizzle half of the spice mixture over the potatoes and toss gently to coat.
4. Bake for 10 minutes.
5. Toss the sweet potatoes with the remaining spice mixture. Add them to the partially cooked baking potatoes and continue baking for 15 minutes more.

Sweet potatoes are not really potatoes, they belong to the 'morning glory' family. Ordinary potatoes are members of the 'nightshade' family. They both can be baked or roasted but sweet potatoes cook faster and will burn if cooked for the same length of time.

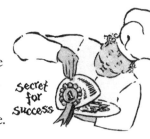

Secret for Success

Makes 4 servings.
Exchanges for each serving of 1/4th recipe:
2 Starch
1/2 Fat

32g Carbohydrate, 4g Protein, 5g Fat, 183 cal
(32g available Carbohydrates)

Potato Corn Cakes

2 cups	Potatoes, boiled & shredded
4	Green onions, chopped
2	Egg whites
1	Egg
1 cup	Frozen corn, thawed
1/4 cup	Red peppers, chopped
1/2 cup	'Light' Cheddar cheese, grated
1/2 tsp	Salt
1/2 tsp	Pepper

1. In a medium mixing bowl combine shredded potatoes, green onions, egg, egg whites, corn, red pepper, grated cheese, salt, & pepper. Divide into eight equal portions. Gently flatten into 3" pancakes and set aside on wax paper while heating pan.
2. Lightly coat a large non-stick frypan or griddle with cooking spray and warm over medium-low heat.
3. Working in two batches add four pancakes at a time to pan. Cook 7 - 8 minutes, turning once, until golden on both sides and cooked through.
4. Remove from pan and keep warm. Respray pan and add remaining batter to make four more pancakes.
5. Serve immediately, topped with 'no fat' sour cream and salsa if desired.

Makes 4 servings.
Exchanges for each serving of 2 potato cakes:
2 Starch
1 Lean meat

32g Carbohydrate, 11g Protein, 4g Fat, 219 cal
(32g available Carbohydrates)

Scalloped Potatoes & Carrots

2 lbs	Potatoes, thinly sliced
2 tbsp	Butter
2 tbsp	All purpose flour
1 1/3 cups	Milk, 1%
1/2 tsp	Salt
1 tsp	Pepper
3/4 cup	'Light' Swiss cheese, grated
1	Egg, beaten
1/4 cup	Onions, diced
3	Carrots, sliced
2 cups	Spinach, chopped
1 tsp	Nutmeg

1. Preheat oven to 350°F. Lightly coat a 9" casserole dish with cooking spray. Peel and thinly slice potatoes into a large bowl of cold salted water. Set aside while preparing the sauce.
2. Melt butter in a small saucepan over medium heat. Whisk in flour. Add milk, salt, & pepper. Cook, stirring constantly until thickened, about 5 mins. Remove from heat, stir in grated cheese. Let cool slightly, then stir in egg.
3. Drain potatoes & pat dry. Layer a third of potatoes in prepared casserole dish. Top with half of onions, carrots & spinach. Sprinkle with nutmeg. Repeat layers. Top with last third of potatoes. Pour sauce evenly over all.
4. Bake uncovered for 1 1/4hrs until potatoes are cooked and top is browned.

Makes 6 servings.
Exchanges for each serving of 1/6th recipe:

2 Starch	1/2 Medium-fat meat
1 Vegetable	1 Fat

36g Carbohydrate, 12g Protein, 8g Fat, 276 cal
(36g available Carbohydrates)

Potato Croquette Casserole

2 lbs	Potatoes (Idaho or russet)
1 tsp	Butter
1/2 cup	Onions, chopped
2 cloves	Garlic, minced
1/2 cup	'Light' sour cream
1/2 cup	'Light' Cheddar cheese, grated
1 tsp	Salt
1/2 tsp	Pepper
1/4 tsp	Nutmeg
1 cup	Breadcrumbs
1/2 cup	Slivered almonds, toasted
2 tbsp	Butter

1. Peel potatoes, cut into quarters and place in a medium sized saucepan. Cover with water, sprinkle with salt. Bring to a boil, reduce heat to simmer and cook for 25 minutes, or until tender. Drain very well. Mash.
2. In a small non-stick frypan, melt 1 tsp butter. Add onion and garlic. Cook until tender. Beat in to mashed potatoes along with sour cream, cheese, salt, pepper, & nutmeg.
3. In a small bowl combine breadcrumbs, almonds, & 2 Tbsp butter.
4. Lightly coat an 9" casserole dish with cooking spray. Spoon in the potato mixture. Sprinkle the crumb mixture on top.
5. Bake at 350°F for 30 minutes.

Make it Special

This elegant side dish is a great choice for a special dinner because it can be assembled early in the day and baked just before serving .

Makes 8 servings.
Exchanges for each serving of 1/8th recipe:

2 Starch	1 Fat
1/2 Vegetable	

32g Carbohydrate, 8g Protein, 9g Fat, 247 cal
(32g available Carbohydrates)

Cauliflower & Broccoli au Gratin

1 lg head	Broccoli, cut in florets
1 lg head	Cauliflower, cut in florets
1 tbsp	Butter
1/4 cup	Onion, chopped
1 tbsp	All purpose flour
1/2 cup	Bread crumbs
3/4 cup	'Light' Cheddar cheese, grated
1 cup	Milk, 1%

1. Cook broccoli and cauliflower until tender crisp by steaming in a saucepan or in the microwave. Immediately rinse with cold water to stop the cooking process. Drain well. Spread in a 9 x 13" casserole dish. Set aside.
2. In a small saucepan melt the butter over medium heat. Cook chopped onion in melted butter for 3 - 4 minutes, just until tender. Stir in flour. Add milk, stir until smooth and thickened. Add salt & pepper. Drizzle over vegetables.
3. Combine bread crumbs and grated cheese, sprinkle evenly over all.
4. Bake at 350°F for 20 to 25 minutes

To steam vegetables in the microwave: wash and then place in a microwave-safe dish. Don't add water, the moisture on the vegetables is enough to steam them. Cover with plastic wrap and cook on high for approximately 4 -5 mins.

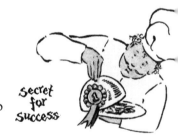

Secret for Success

Makes 8 servings.
Exchanges for each serving of 1/8th recipe:
2 Vegetable   1/2 Fat
1/2 Medium-fat meat

11g Carbohydrate, 8g Protein, 5g Fat, 120 cal
(11 g available Carbohydrates)

Muffins & Breads

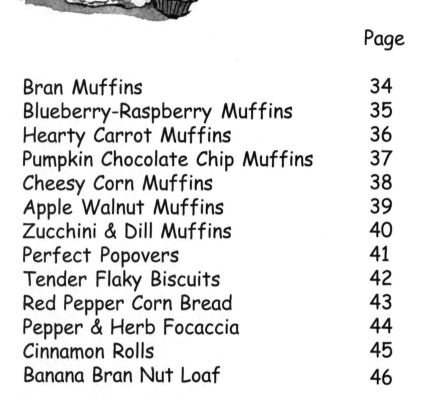

Bran Muffins

1 1/3 cups	Buttermilk, low fat
3/4 cup	All Bran® cereal
3/4 cup	Bran, 100%
2 1/2 cups	All purpose flour
1/2 cup	Splenda®
4 tsp	Baking powder
2 tsp	Baking soda
1/4 tsp	Cinnamon
1/4 tsp	Salt
1/2 cup	Applesauce, unsweetened
1/4 cup	Molasses, light
1 tsp	Vegetable oil
1	Egg
1 tsp	Vanilla extract
1/3 cup	Raisins

1. Preheat oven 375°F. Lightly coat 16 muffin cups with cooking spray or line with paper liners.
2. In a large mixing bowl combine buttermilk with All Bran® and 100% bran. Let stand for 10 minutes. In a separate bowl, stir together the flour, Splenda®, baking powder, baking soda, cinnamon & salt.
3. Stir applesauce, molasses, vegetable oil, egg & vanilla into the bran mixture. Mix well. Make a well in the center of the flour mixture, pour in the applesauce/bran mixture and currants. Stir just until combined.
4. Spoon batter into prepared muffin cups. Bake for 25 minutes.

Makes 16 servings.
Exchanges for each serving of 1 muffin:

1 Starch	1/2 Fat
1 Fruit	

27g Carbohydrate, 4g protein, 4g Fat, 169 cal
(27g available Carbohydrates)

Blueberry-Raspberry Muffins

1 cup	All purpose flour
1 cup	Whole wheat flour
1/2 cup	Cornmeal
1/2 cup	Splenda®
2 tsp	Baking powder
1 tsp	Baking soda
1/4 tsp	Salt
1/4 cup	Cold margarine, diced
3/4 cup	Plain yogurt, low fat
1/2 cup	Orange juice
2	Eggs
3/4 cup	Blueberries, fresh or frozen
3/4 cup	Raspberries, fresh or frozen

1. Preheat oven to 400°F. Lightly coat 16 muffin cups with cooking spray or line with paper liners.
2. In a large bowl combine flours, cornmeal, Splenda®, baking powder, baking soda, and salt. With 2 knives, cut in margarine until mixture is crumb like.
3. In a small mixing bowl combine yogurt, orange juice, & eggs.
4. Make a well in the center of the dry ingredients and pour in egg mixture. Stir just until combined. Gently fold in blueberries & raspberries.
5. Fill muffin cups 2/3 full. Bake 18-20 min or until golden.

chef's secret...

To freeze berries so they don't stick together: arrange dry berries in a single layer on a baking sheet; freeze 2 hours. Transfer to a freezer bag.

Makes 16 servings.
Exchanges for each serving of 1 muffin:
1 Starch
1/2 Fat

18g Carbohydrate, 4g Protein, 4g Fat, 122 cal
(18g available Carbohydrates)

Hearty Carrot Muffins

2 cups	All Bran® cereal
1 1/4 cups	Buttermilk, low fat
1/3 cup	Vegetable oil
2	Eggs
3	Carrots, shredded
1/2 cup	Coconut, unsweetened
1/2 cup	Raisins
1 1/4 cups	All purpose flour
1/3 cup	Brown sugar
1/4 cup	Splenda®
2 tsp	Baking powder
1 tsp	Baking soda
1 tsp	Cinnamon
1/2 tsp	Salt

1. Preheat oven to 375°F. Lightly coat 18 muffin cups with cooking spray or line with paper liners
2. In a large mixing bowl combine All Bran®, buttermilk, oil, & eggs. Let stand for 10 minutes. Stir in carrot, coconut & raisins.
3. In a separate mixing bowl combine flour, sugar, Splenda®, baking powder, baking soda, cinnamon, & salt. Make a well in the center of the dry ingredients. Add cereal mixture, stir just until combined.
4. Fill prepared muffin cups 2/3 full. Bake for 20 minutes.

Makes 18 servings.
Exchanges for each serving of 1 muffin:
1 Starch   1 Fat
1 Vegetable

19g Carbohydrate, 4g Protein, 7g Fat, 151 cal
(19g available Carbohydrates)

Pumpkin Chocolate Chip Muffins

2 cups	All purpose flour
1/2 cup	Splenda®
1/4 cup	Brown sugar
1 tbsp	Baking powder
1 tsp	Cinnamon
1 tsp	Ginger, ground
1/4 tsp	Salt
3/4 cup	Pumpkin, canned or cooked
1	Egg
2/3 cup	Milk, 1%
3 tbsp	Vegetable oil
1 tsp	Vanilla extract
1/3 cup	Mini chocolate chips

1. Preheat oven to 375°F. Coat 12 muffin cups with cooking spray.
2. In a large mixing bowl combine flour, Splenda®, brown sugar, baking powder, and spices.
3. In a separate mixing bowl beat together the pumpkin, egg, milk, oil, and vanilla. Make a well in the center of the dry ingredients, pour in the pumpkin mixture. Stir just until combined. Gently fold in the chocolate chips.
4. Spoon into prepared muffin cups and bake for 25 minutes.

healthy hint...

Using fruit or vegetable purees in baking (such as pumpkin), allows you to use less fats while retaining moisture and flavor.

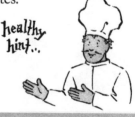

Makes 12 servings.
Exchanges for each serving of 1 muffin

1 Starch	1 Fat
1 Fruit	

27g Carbohydrate, 4g Protein, 6g Fat, 176 cal
(27g available Carbohydrates)

Cheesy Corn Muffins

1 1/2 cups	Cornmeal
1 cup	All purpose flour
2 tbsp	Splenda®
1 tbsp	Baking powder
1/2 tsp	Salt
3	Eggs
1 1/2 cups	Buttermilk, low fat
1 1/3 cups	Corn kernels, (frozen & thawed or canned & drained)
3/4 cup	'Light' Cheddar cheese, grated
4	Green onions, chopped
1/4 cup	Vegetable oil

1. Preheat oven to 400°F. Lightly coat 15 muffin cups with cooking spray.
2. Mix cornmeal, flour, Splenda®, baking powder, & salt in a large bowl.
3. In a separate bowl beat eggs lightly with a fork. Stir in buttermilk, corn, grated cheese, green onions & vegetable oil. Pour liquid mixture all at once into dry ingredients, stir with a fork just until mixed (batter will be lumpy).
4. Fill muffin cups three-quarters full with batter. Bake for 25 minutes or until golden brown. Best served warm from the oven.

chef's secret...

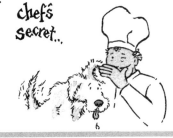

Spray the bottoms of the muffin cups only, spraying the sides stops the tops from rounding nicely.

Makes 15 servings.
Exchanges for each serving of 1 muffin:
1 1/2 Starch   1/2 Fat
1/2 Medium-fat meat

21g Carbohydrate, 6g Protein, 6g Fat, 170 cal
(22 g available Carbohydrates)

Apple Walnut Muffins

2 cups	All purpose flour
1 tbsp	Baking powder
1 tsp	Cinnamon
1/2 tsp	Salt
1	Egg
1 1/4 cups	Milk, 1%
1/4 cup	White sugar
1/4 cup	Brown sugar
1/4 cup	Vegetable oil
1 tsp	Vanilla extract
2	Apples, peeled & grated
1/4 cup	Walnuts, chopped

1. Preheat oven to 400°F. Lightly coat 12 muffin cups with cooking spray or line with paper liners.
2. In a large mixing bowl combine the flour, baking powder, cinnamon, & salt.
3. In a separate bowl beat the egg, milk, sugars, vegetable oil, & vanilla.
4. Make a well in dry ingredients. Pour in egg mixture along with the grated apple and walnuts. Stir just until mixed. Spoon into prepared muffin cups.
5. Bake for 20 minutes or until tops spring back when lightly touched.

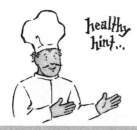

healthy hint... Cut down on the saturated fats in your diet by substituting vegetable oil in recipes that call for melted butter.

Makes 12 servings.
Exchanges for each serving of 1 muffin:
1 1/2 Starch   1 Fat
1/2 Fruit

28g Carbohydrate, 4g Protein, 7g Fat, 195cal
(28g available Carbohydrates)

Zucchini & Dill Muffins

1 3/4 cups	All purpose flour
1 tbsp	Baking powder
1 tsp	Salt
1	Egg
1/4 cup	White sugar
3/4 cup	Milk, 1%
1/4 cup	Vegetable oil
1 tsp	Dill weed, dried
1 cup	Zucchini, shredded
1/4 cup	Parmesan cheese, grated

1. Preheat oven to 400°F. Coat 12 muffin cups with cooking spray.
2. Combine flour, baking powder, and salt in a large mixing bowl.
3. In a separate mixing bowl beat eggs, sugar, milk, vegetable oil & dill. Stir in grated zucchini.
4. Pour egg mixture all at once into dry ingredients, stir just until all ingredients are moistened. Batter will look lumpy, do not overstir.
5. Fill muffin cups 3/4 full with batter. Sprinkle tops with parmesan cheese.
6. Bake for 25 minutes or until golden brown. Best served hot from the oven.

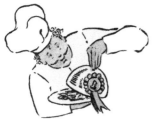

Secret for Success!

Don't try to use paper liners for this recipe. They become nearly impossible to peel off!

Makes 12 servings.
Exchanges for each serving of 1 muffin:

1 Starch	1 Fat
1 Vegetable	

19g Carbohydrate, 4g Protein, 5g Fat, 143 cal
(19g available Carbohydrates)

Perfect Popovers

2	Egg whites
1	Egg
1 cup	Milk, 1%
1 tbsp	Vegetable oil
1 cup	All purpose flour
1/2 tsp	Salt

1. Preheat oven to 400°F. Coat 10 large muffin cups with cooking spray.
2. Beat egg whites and egg together with an electric mixer until frothy. Beat
 in milk and vegetable oil. Add flour and salt, continue to beat until blended.
3. Fill prepared muffin cups half full. Bake for 30 - 35 minutes, until firm.
4. Turn off oven. Prick popovers with a fork and leave in warm oven for
 8 to10 minutes to crisp. Serve warm.

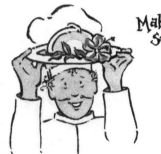

Make it Special

Use a popover pan (or 6 custard cups) to make 6 large popovers instead of 10 smaller ones. They may be used as a shell for main dishes such as Chicken a la King (pg.66).

Makes 10 servings.
Exchanges for each serving of 1 popover:
1/2 Starch   1/2 Fat
1/2 Vegetable

10g Carbohydrate, 3g protein, 2g fat, 79 cal
(10g available Carbohydrates)

Tender Flaky Biscuits

2 cups	Cake flour
2 tsp	Baking powder
1/4 tsp	Baking soda
1/4 tsp	Salt
1/4 cup	Cold margarine, diced
3/4 cup	Buttermilk, low fat

1. Preheat oven to 450°F.
2. In a medium mixing bowl combine flour, baking powder, baking soda, and salt. Cut in margarine with a pastry blender until lumps are pea-sized or smaller. Stir in buttermilk with a fork. Press dough into a ball.
3. On a lightly floured surface roll dough into a 6 x 10" rectangle. Fold in short ends to meet in the center. Fold dough in half so it is four layers thick. Roll dough into 6" square.
4. With a floured knife cut into 12 squares. Place 1 1/2" apart on an ungreased baking sheet. Bake 10 -12 minutes, until lightly browned.

chef's secret...

for tender biscuits...
✔ Use cake flour ✔ Use margarine instead of butter ✔ Fold dough to increase flakiness ✔ Handle the dough as little as possible.

time for a change

cheese biscuits...
Stir 1/2 cup shredded cheddar & 2 Tbsp chopped chives or green onions in with the buttermilk.

Makes 12 servings.
Exchanges for each serving of 1 biscuit:
1 Starch
1/2 Fat

1 Cheese Biscuit:
1 Starch
1 Fat
16g carbohydrate, 4g protein,5 g fat, 121 cal

15g Carbohydrate, 2g Protein, 4g Fat, 107 cal
(15g available Carbohydrates)

Red Pepper Corn Bread

1 1/2 cups	Cornmeal
1/2 cup	All purpose flour
2 tbsp	Splenda®
2 tsp	Baking powder
1 tsp	Baking soda
1 tsp	Cumin
1/4 tsp	Pepper
1 tsp	Salt
1 1/2 cups	Buttermilk, low fat
2	Eggs
2 tbsp	Vegetable oil
1	Red pepper, diced

1 Preheat oven to 425°F. Lightly coat a 9" square baking pan with cooking spray.
2. Combine the first eight ingredients in a large mixing bowl. With an electric mixer, beat the buttermilk, egg, & oil together in a separate mixing bowl.
3. Add egg mixture to dry ingredients along with the diced red pepper, stir just until blended.
4. Spread in the prepared pan and bake 25 - 30 minutes, until firm.
5. Cut into 16 squares and serve warm.

Makes 16 servings.
Exchanges for each serving of 1 square:
1 Starch
1/2 Fat

15g Carbohydrate, 3g Protein, 3g Fat, 100 cal
(15g available Carbohydrates)

Pepper & Herb Focaccia

2 cups	Bread flour
1 tbsp	Yeast, 'rapid rise'
1 tsp	Salt
1 1/2 tsp	White sugar
2 tbsp	Cornmeal
2 tbsp	Olive oil
6	Green onions, chopped
2 tsp	Rosemary, dried
1 tsp	Thyme, dried
1/2 tsp	Sage, dried
1/2 tsp	Pepper
1/4 tsp	Cayenne pepper

1. Blend flour, yeast, salt, & sugar in a food processor. Combine 3/4 cup hot tap water and 1Tbsp olive oil. With machine running, pour water mixture through feed tube. Process until the dough forms a ball, about 40 seconds. Coat the surface of the ball with cooking spray and transfer to an oiled bowl. Cover with a damp towel and let rise for 30 minutes.
2. Punch dough down. Knead until smooth. Cover and let rest for 10 minutes.
3. Heat 1 tsp olive oil in a small frypan over medium heat. Add green onions, herbs, and spices. Saute until fragrant and onion is softened.
4. Lightly coat a baking sheet with cooking spray. Sprinkle with cornmeal.
5. Roll out dough on a lightly floured surface to a 12" round. Place on prepared pan. Dimple suface with a wooden spoon handle. Spread with remaining olive oil and sprinkle with herb mixture. Let rise 30 minutes.
6. Preheat oven to 400°F. Bake 20 minutes, until golden.

Makes 14 servings.
Exchanges for each serving of 1 wedge:
1 Starch
1/2 Fat

17g Carbohydrate, 3g Protein, 2g Fat, 99 cal
(17g available Carbohydrates)

Cinnamon Rolls

1 lb	Frozen Bread dough
2 tbsp	Butter, melted
1/4 cup	Brown sugar
1 tbsp	Cinnamon
1/2 cup	Raisins (or currants)
3 tbsp	Confectioner's sugar
3 tbsp	Orange juice, freshly squeezed

1. Thaw dough and let rise. Punch dough down. On a lightly floured surface, roll dough into a 14 x 10" rectangle. Brush with melted butter.
2. In a small bowl stir together brown sugar, & cinnamon. Sprinkle sugar mixture and raisins evenly over the dough.
3. Beginning at narrow end, roll up tightly. Pinch seam to seal. Cut into 16 equal slices.
4. Place cut sides up in a 9 x 13" baking pan that has been coated with cooking spray. Cover and let rise until doubled in size, 45 minutes.
5. Preheat oven to 375°F. Bake for 15 -20 minutes or until golden brown.
6. Combine icing sugar and orange juice, drizzle over warm rolls.

Makes 16 servings.
Exchanges for each serving of 1 roll:
1 Starch   1/2 Fat
1/2 Fruit

21g Carbohydrate, 2g Protein, 3g Fat, 121 cal
(21g available Carbohydrates)

Banana Bran Nut Loaf

1/4 cup	Margarine, softened
1	Egg
1 cup	All Bran® cereal
2 cups	Bananas, mashed
1/2 cup	Walnuts, chopped
1 tsp	Vanilla extract
1 1/2 cups	All purpose flour
1/4 cup	Splenda®
2 tsp	Baking powder
1/2 tsp	Baking soda
1/2 tsp	Salt
1/2 cup	Dried apricots, chopped

1. Preheat oven to 350°F. Lightly coat a 9 x 5" loaf pan with cooking spray.
2. In a large mixing bowl, cream margarine with an electric mixer. Add egg and continue beating until well mixed. Add All Bran®, mashed banana, walnuts & vanilla; beat until smooth.
3. In a separate bowl stir together the flour, Splenda®, baking powder, baking soda & salt. Add to margarine mixture along with the chopped apricots. Stir just until mixed.
4. Spoon into the prepared loaf pan and bake for 50 - 60 minutes.
5. Allow to cool on a wire rack. Cut into 16 slices to serve.

Makes 16 servings
Exchanges for each serving of 1 slice:
1 Starch   1 Fat
1/2 Fruit

20g Carbohydrate, 4g Protein, 5g fat, 143 cal
(20g available Carbohydrates)

Breakfast & Brunch

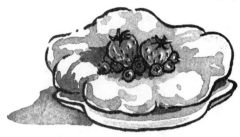

Breakfast in a Bun

4	Eggs
2	Egg whites
4	Green onions, chopped
1	Tomato, chopped
1/2 tsp	Salt
1/2 tsp	Pepper
4 oz	Turkey ham, thinly sliced
4	English muffins
1/2 cup	'Light' Cheddar cheese, grated

1. With a fork beat the eggs and egg whites until well combined. Stir in the chopped green onions, tomatoes, salt & pepper.
2. Lightly coat a non-stick frypan with cooking spray and heat over medium heat. Add turkey ham slices and fry just until hot and edges begin to crisp. Remove from the pan.
3. Respray pan with cooking spray and add egg mixture. Cook, stirring occasionally, until set and cooked through.
4. While eggs are cooking toast English muffins under the broiler..
5. Place a slice of turkey ham on each English muffin bottom. Top with scrambled egg mixture & grated cheese. Return to broiler and cook just until cheese melts, 2-3 mins.
6. Replace top halves of muffins and serve.

Makes 4 servings.
Exchanges for each serving of 1 Breakfast Bun:
2 Starch
3 Lean meat

31g Carbohydrate, 25g Protein, 11g Fat, 328 cal
(31g available Carbohydrates)

Overnight Egg Scramble

1 tbsp	Butter, divided
1 tbsp	All purpose flour
1 cup	Milk, 1%
1 cup	'Light' Cheddar cheese, grated
2 cups	Broccoli, chopped
2 cups	Mushrooms, sliced
6	Green onions, chopped
4	Eggs
4	Egg whites
1/2 tsp	Salt
1/2 tsp	Pepper
2/3 cup	Breadcrumbs

1. In a small saucepan melt 2 tsp butter over medium heat. Add flour; cook and stir until mixture bubbles. Whisk in milk, bring to a boil. Cook and stir until smooth & thickened. Stir in half of the cheese. Set aside.
2. Microwave or steam broccoli until tender crisp, 3-4 mins. Drain well.
3. Lightly coat a large frypan with cooking spray. Add 1 tsp butter & heat over medium-high heat. Add mushrooms & onions, saute until tender, 3-4 mins.
4. Meanwhile stir together the eggs, egg whites, salt & pepper. Add to frypan, cook and stir until the eggs are set. Stir in cooked broccoli.
5. Lightly coat a 12 x 8" casserole dish with cooking spray. Spoon in egg mixture, pour cheese sauce over and toss gently to coat. Sprinkle with remaining cheese & breadcrumbs. Cover & refrigerate overnight.
6. Uncover and bake at 350°F for 30 mins.

Makes 6 servings.
Each serving of 1/6th recipe:
1 Starch
2 Medium-fat meat

16g Carbohydrate, 17g Protein, 10g Fat, 231 cal
(15g available Carbohydrates)

Eggs "Benny"

3 1/2 oz	'Light' cream cheese
1/4 cup	Plain yogurt, low fat
2 tsp	Lemon juice
1 tsp	Dijon mustard
4	Eggs
8 slices	Canadian back bacon
2	English muffins (4 halves)
8 large	Spinach leaves, washed
1/2	Red pepper, thinly sliced

1. Combine cream cheese, yogurt, lemon juice, and mustard in a small saucepan over low heat. Stir with a whisk while heating gently, until smooth. Keep warm while preparing eggs. Do not allow to boil.

2. To poach eggs: bring a large pot of water (6 cups) to boil. Reduce heat to simmer. Break an egg into a small bowl and slide into the water. Repeat with remaining 3 eggs. Simmer for about 5 minutes, until yolks are just set. Carefully lift from water with a slotted spoon.

3. Meanwhile lightly fry back bacon and toast English muffins.

4. Top each muffin half with 2 spinach leaves, 2 slices of bacon & 1 egg. Spoon sauce over eggs, garnish with red pepper slices & serve.

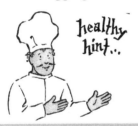

healthy hint... For a meatless version you can substitute 'Canadian Veggie Bacon®'. The results are equally tasty and slightly lower in fat.

Makes 4 servings.
Exchanges for each serving of one egg topped muffin:
1 Starch
3 Medium-fat meat

17g Carbohydrate, 24g protein, 14g fat, 306 cal
(17g available Carbohydrates)

Huevos Rancheros

4	8" Whole wheat tortillas
4	Eggs
1/2 cup	Salsa
1/2 tsp	Salt
1/2 tsp	Pepper
3/4 cup	'Light' Cheddar cheese, grated
6	Green onions, chopped
6	Radishes, sliced

Mock Guacamole:

1 clove	Garlic, minced
2/3 cup	Frozen peas, thawed
2 tbsp	Cilantro, snipped
1 tsp	Lemon juice
1/4 tsp	Tabasco Sauce

1. Make guacamole by processing all ingredients in a food processor until smooth. Preheat oven to 350°F.
2. Arrange tortillas in a single layer on a baking sheet. Spray lightly with cooking spray and bake 8-10 minutes, until crisp and toasted.
3. Lightly coat a non-stick frypan with cooking spray. Carefully break eggs into pan. Spoon salsa around eggs, sprinkle with salt & pepper. Cover and cook until whites are set and yolks are jiggly.
4. Place toasted tortillas on serving plates, top each with 1/4 of the cheese, a fried egg & salsa, green onions, radishes, and mock guacamole (if desired).

Makes 4 servings.
Exchanges for each serving of 1 Huevo Ranchero:
1 1/2 Starch
2 Medium-fat meat

25g Carbohydrate, 18g Protein, 12g Fat, 276 cal
(25g available Carbohydrates)

Farmer's Casserole

2 lbs	Baking potatoes (5 medium)
1 cup	'Light' Cheddar cheese, grated
6 slices	Bacon, cooked & crumbled
6	Green onions, chopped
1	Red pepper, chopped
6	Eggs
1	can (12oz) Evaporated skim milk
1/4 tsp	Pepper

1. Peel potatoes, cut into even sized pieces and place in a medium-sized saucepan. Cover with water and bring to a boil; reduce heat. Simmer for 20 -25 mins, until just tender. Allow to cool.
2. Lightly coat a 9 x 13" baking dish with cooking spray. Coarsley shred potatoes and spread in prepared pan. Sprinkle with cheese, bacon, green onions, & red peppers.
3. In a medium-sized bowl beat together the eggs, evaporated skim milk & pepper. Pour over casserole. Cover and refrigerate several hours or overnight.
4. Preheat oven to 350°F. Uncover casserole and bake for 55 - 60 minutes, or until firm.

chefs secret...

You can make this recipe faster by using 'store-bought' hashbrowns. Try one of the fresh grated variety with no added fat.

Makes 6 servings.
Exchanges for each serving of 1/6th recipe:

1 Starch	1 Vegetable
1 Low-fat milk	1 High-fat meat

36g Carbohydrate, 21g Protein, 12g Fat, 328 cal
(36g available Carbohydrates)

Corned Beef Hash Frittata

1 lb	Frozen hash brown potatoes, unprepared
1/2 cup	Onions, diced
1	Red or green pepper, diced
1	can (7oz) Corned beef
4	Eggs
4	Egg whites
1/2 tsp	Pepper
1/2 cup	'Light' Cheddar cheese, grated

1. Lightly coat a large non-stick frypan with cooking spray and heat over medium heat.
2. Add hash brown potatoes, onions, & peppers; cook for 8 - 10 mins., stirring occasionally. Flake corned beef with a fork and add to potato mixture. Continue cooking for 5 -7 mins, until potatoes are golden and onion is tender.
3. Meanwhile, in a medium-sized mixing bowl beat eggs, whites, & pepper together with a fork.
4. Reduce heat to low; pour eggs over potato mixture. Cover and cook 6 - 8 minutes, until eggs are set.
5. Sprinkle with grated cheese. Cut into 6 wedges and serve.

Instead of corned beef try cooked & crumbled 'low-fat' Italian sausage or canned "Flakes of ham or turkey". This recipe is a favorite for camping!

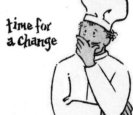

time for a change

Makes 6 servings.
Exchanges for each serving of 1 wedge:
1 Starch
3 Lean meat

16g Carbohydrate, 20g Protein, 10g Fat, 242 cal
(16g available Carbohydrates)

"No Crust" Quiche

1 1/2 cups	Broccoli, chopped
1/4 cup	Onions, chopped
1 cup	Lean ham (5% fat), diced
1 1/2 cups	'Light' Cheddar cheese, grated
3	Eggs
6	Egg whites
1/2 cup	Milk, 1%
1/4 cup	'Light' mayonnaise
1/2 tsp	Salt
1/2 tsp	Pepper
1/4 cup	Parmesan cheese, grated

1. Preheat oven to 375°F. Lightly coat a 9" pie plate with cooking spray.
2. Place chopped broccoli & onions in a microwave safe casserole, cover with plastic wrap and microwave on high for 3-4 mins, until tender crisp. Rinse immediately with cold water to stop cooking and retain bright color. Drain.
3. Combine broccoli, onions, ham & cheddar cheese in prepared pie plate.
4. In a large mixing bowl whisk together eggs, egg whites, milk, mayonnaise, salt & pepper. Pour over broccoli mixture. Sprinkle with parmesan cheese.
5. Bake 40 minutes or until firm. Cut into 6 wedges to serve.

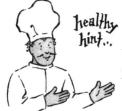

healthy hint...

Using egg whites or egg substitute instead of whole eggs?
2 egg whites or 1/4 cup egg substitute = 1 whole egg.

Makes 6 servings.
Exchanges for each serving of 1 wedge:
1 Vegetable
3 Medium-fat meat

6g Carbohydrate, 23g Protein, 13g Fat, 242 cal
(6g available Carbohydrates)

Cheese & Veggie Strata

2 cups	Mushrooms, sliced
1	Red or green peppers, diced
6	Green onions, chopped
2 cloves	Garlic, minced
4	Eggs
4	Egg whites
1 1/3 cups	Milk, 1%
1/2 tsp	Salt
1/4 tsp	Pepper
8 slices	Whole-wheat bread, cubed
1 1/4 cups	'Light' Cheddar cheese, grated

1. Lightly coat a 9 x 13" casserole dish with cooking spray and set aside.
2. Coat a large non-stick frypan with cooking spray; heat over medium heat. Add mushrooms, peppers, onions, and garlic. Stir fry until tender, 5 - 6 mins.
3. In a large mixing bowl beat the eggs, egg whites, milk, salt & pepper.
4. Spread half of the bread cubes over the bottom of the prepared casserole dish. Spoon half of the mushroom mixture over the bread cubes and sprinkle with half of the cheese. Repeat the layers ending with the cheese.
5. Pour the egg mixture over all, being sure to coat all the bread cubes. (May be covered & refrigerated overnight at this point).
6. Preheat oven to 350°F. Bake, uncovered 40 mins; until puffed and golden.

Makes 6 servings.
Exchanges for each serving of 1/6th recipe:
1 Starch   2 Medium-fat meat
1 Vegetable

20g Carbohydrate, 20g Protein, 10g fat, 254 cal
(20g available Carbohydrates)

Buckwheat & Fruit Pancakes

1 cup	Buckwheat flour
1 cup	Whole wheat flour
2 tbsp	Splenda®
2 tsp	Baking powder
1/2 tsp	Baking soda
1 cup	Buttermilk, low fat
1 cup	Plain yogurt, low fat
1/2 cup	Applesauce, unsweetened
2	Egg whites
2 cups	Blueberries

1. Combine first five ingredients in a large mixing bowl.

2. In a separate mixing bowl stir together buttermilk, yogurt, applesauce, & egg whites. Stir buttermilk mixture into dry ingredients, along with blueberries. Stir just until blended.

3. Lightly coat a large non-stick frypan or griddle with cooking spray and heat over medium heat.

4. When pan is hot, pour batter by quarter cupfuls into frypan. Cook until bubbles appear on surface, flip and continue cooking until golden brown.

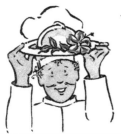

Make it Special

Use any fresh seasonal berries or chopped fruit instead of blueberries.

Makes 6 servings.
Exchanges for each serving of 3 pancakes:
2 Starch   1/2 Skim milk
1/2 Fruit

43g Carbohydrate, 10g Protein, 2g Fat, 228 cal
(43g available Carbohydrates)

Peachy Pancakes

1 1/4 cups	Rolled oats, quick or regular
2 cups	Buttermilk, low fat
1	Egg
1/4 cup	Applesauce, unsweetened
1 tsp	Vanilla extract
1 cup	All purpose flour
1/4 cup	Wheat germ, toasted
2 tbsp	Splenda®
1 tbsp	Baking powder
1/2 tsp	Salt
1/2 tsp	Cinnamon
2	Peaches, peeled & diced
	(or 7oz 'juice packed' canned peaches)

1. Mix oats & buttermilk. Let stand 10 mins. Stir in egg, applesauce, & vanilla.
2. In a separate mixing bowl combine flour, wheat germ, Splenda®, baking powder, salt & cinnamon. Add dry ingredients to oat mixture and stir until blended. Gently fold in diced peaches.
3. Coat a non-stick griddle or frypan with cooking spray. Heat to medium-hot.
4. For each pancake; pour 1/4 cup batter onto hot griddle. Cook, turning once, until golden brown and cooked through. Makes 15 pancakes.

This pancake batter is great for weekend camping or skiing trips because it can be made the night before.

Makes 5 servings.
Exchanges for each serving of 3 pancakes.

2 Starch	1/2 Low-fat milk
1/2 Fruit	

44g Carbohydrate, 12g Protein, 4g Fat, 277 cal
(44g available Carbohydrates)

Overnight French Toast

1 tbsp	Butter
12 slices	French or Vienna bread
1 cup	Milk, 1%
1/4 cup	Splenda®
2 tbsp	Pure Maple syrup
1 tsp	Vanilla extract
1/2 tsp	Salt
4	Egg whites
4	Eggs

1. Spread butter over a heavy baking sheet (or cookie sheet) with 1" sides. Arrange bread slices on buttered pan in a single layer.
2. Beat eggs, egg whites, milk, Splenda®, maple syrup, vanilla, & salt in a large mixing bowl.
3. Pour egg mixture over bread. Cover with plastic wrap and refrigerate overnight.
4. Preheat oven 400°F. Bake French toast, uncovered, for 10 minutes. Flip bread slices over and continue baking for 5 minutes.

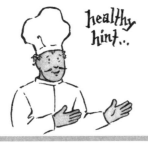

healthy hint...

Pure maple syrup is intensely flavored. Therefore a small amount adds a lot of flavor and keeps the sugar content low.

Makes 6 servings.
Exchanges for each serving of 2 slices:

2 Starch	1/2 Medium-fat meat
1/2 Low-fat milk	

34g Carbohydrate, 12g Protein, 7g Fat, 257 cal
(34 g available Carbohydrates)

Monte Cristo Sandwiches

2	Eggs
1/4 cup	Milk, 1%
1/2 tsp	Salt
1/2 tsp	Pepper
8 slices	French bread
4 oz	'Light' Swiss cheese, sliced
6 oz	Lean cooked ham, thinly sliced
4 tsp	Dijon mustard

1. Preheat oven to 425°F. Lightly coat a cookie sheet with cooking spray.
2. In a shallow bowl or pie plate beat eggs, milk, salt and pepper with a fork.
3. Put sliced cheese on each of 4 slices of bread, top with ham. Spread Dijon mustard on the other 4 slices of bread. Place mustard side down on ham.
4. Dip both sides of sandwich in egg mixture. Place on prepared cookie sheet.
5. Bake 15 -18 minutes turning once, until both sides are browned and the cheese is melted.

time for a change

Make 'Italian' sandwiches by using pesto instead of Dijon mustard and Mozzarella or Provolone cheese instead of Swiss. Turkey can be substituted for some or all of the ham.

Makes 4 servings.
Exchanges for each serving of 1 sandwich:
2 Starch
3 Lean meat

30g Carbohydrate, 26g Protein, 8g Fat, 322 cal
(30g available Carbohydrates)

Fruity Clafouti

3	Eggs
1 1/4 cups	Milk, 1%
2/3 cup	All purpose flour
1/4 cup	Splenda®
2 tsp	Vanilla extract
1/4 tsp	Nutmeg, ground
1/4 tsp	Salt
1 1/2 cups	Raspberries, fresh or frozen (thawed)
2	Kiwi, sliced & halved

1. Preheat oven to 350°F. Lightly coat a 9" quiche dish or pie plate with butter flavored cooking spray.
2. In a medium sized mixing bowl beat eggs with an electric mixer until foamy. Add milk, flour, Splenda®, vanilla, nutmeg, & salt. Beat on low, until smooth.
3. Pour into prepared baking dish. Sprinkle with raspberries, & kiwi, reserving a few for garnish.
4. Bake for 40 -45 minutes, until a knife inserted in the centre comes out clean. Let stand for 15 minutes. Garnish with reserved fruit and serve.

Make it Special

This countrified French pancake is traditionally made with cherries but it can be made with any fresh seasonal fruit. It can be served for breakfast or topped with whipped cream & served for dessert.

Makes 8 servings.
Exchanges for each serving of 1 wedge:
1/2 Starch   1/2 Medium-fat meat
1/2 Fruit

15g Carbohydrate, 5g Protein, 3g Fat, 111 cal
(15g available Carbohydrates)

Poultry

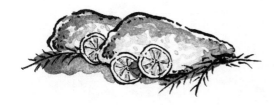

Ginger Orange Chicken

4 halves (1 lb)	Chicken breasts, skinless
3/4 cup	Orange juice
1/3 cup	Soy sauce
1 tbsp	Brown sugar
1 tbsp	Splenda®
1 tbsp	Ginger root, grated
1 1/2 tbsp	Cornstarch
1	Orange, sliced
2 tbsp	Parsley, snipped

1. Preheat oven to 350°F. Arrange chicken breasts in a single layer, top side up, in a baking dish.
2. In a small bowl combine orange juice, soy sauce, brown sugar, & ginger. Pour over chicken. Bake for 35 minutes.
3. Remove chicken from the pan. Combine cornstarch with Splenda®, and 1/2 cup of water. Stir until smooth and then stir into pan juices.
4. Put chicken back into the pan, top side down in the sauce. Bake 10 -15 minutes longer or until sauce is thickened and chicken is tender when pierced with a small sharp knife.
5. Garnish with orange slices and parsley.

Makes 4 servings.
Exchanges for each serving of 1 chicken breast:
1 Fruit
4 Very lean meat

16g Carbohydrate, 30g protein, 2g fat, 206kcal (862kJ)
(16g available Carbohydrates)

Chicken Marengo

2 tsp	Olive Oil
4 halves (1 lb)	Chicken breasts, boneless, skinless
1/2 cup	Onions, chopped
2 cups	Mushrooms, sliced
2 cloves	Garlic, minced
1	can (14oz) Stewed tomatoes
1/4 cup	White wine
2 tsp	Rosemary, fresh
2 tbsp	Parsley, fresh, chopped
1/2 tsp	Salt
1/2 tsp	Thyme, dried
1/4 tsp	Pepper

1. Heat olive oil in a large non-stick skillet over medium-high heat. Add chicken and brown, about 4 minutes per side, until golden. Remove from pan.
2. Add onions, mushrooms, & garlic to the pan; saute until tender.
3. Add tomatoes, wine & rosemary. Heat to boiling, reduce heat to simmer and return chicken to the pan.
4. Combine parsley, salt, thyme, & pepper; sprinkle over the chicken. Cover and simmer for 25 - 30 minutes, until chicken is cooked through.

chef's secret...
To use fresh rosemary: strip the leaves from the stem and mince fine. Heat softens the leaves and releases the flavor, so always add rosemary at the start of the cooking process.

Makes 4 servings.
Exchanges for each serving of 1 chicken breast:
1 Starch
4 Very lean meat

13g Carbohydrate, 30g Protein, 4g Fat, 223 cal
(13g available Carbohydrates)

Chicken Piccata

4 halves (1 lb)	Chicken breasts, boneless, skinless
1/2 cup	Onions, chopped
3	Carrots, peeled & sliced diagonally
1	Red pepper, thinly sliced
1/2 tsp	Salt
1/2 tsp	Pepper
1/2 cup	White wine
2 tbsp	Capers
2 tbsp	Butter
2 tbsp	All purpose flour
1/4 cup	Fresh lemon juice

1. Pound chicken breasts between two pieces of wax paper to flatten.
2. Lightly coat a large non-stick skillet with cooking spray. Add onions & carrots and cook over medium heat until almost tender, about 6-8 minutes. Remove from pan.
3. Meanwhile, in a shallow dish or pie plate combine flour with 1/4 tsp salt & pepper. Roll chicken in mixture.
4. Respray pan with cooking spray and heat over med-high heat. Add chicken and cook until brown, turning once, about 3 minutes per side. Return onions & carrots to pan. Add lemon juice, wine, capers, red pepper strips, and remaining salt & pepper. Dot with butter.
5. Cover and simmer for 15 - 20 minutes or until chicken is tender. Serve garnished with chopped parsley and lemon slices.

Makes 4 servings.
Exchanges for each serving of 1 chicken breast:

1/2 Fruit	4 Very lean meat
1 Vegetable	1/2 Fat

11g Carbohydrate, 29g Protein, 7g Fat, 249 cal
(11g available Carbohydrates)

Jamaiican Jerk Chicken

3/4 cup	Vinegar
1/2 cup	Orange juice
1/4 cup	Soy sauce
1/2 cup	Onions, chopped
1/4 cup	Jalapeno peppers, minced
2 tbsp	Lime juice
2 cloves	Garlic, minced
1 tsp	Salt
2 tsp	Thyme, dried
1 tsp	Allspice
1/2 tsp	Tabasco sauce
6 halves (1 1/2lbs)	Chicken breasts

1. Combine all ingredients except chicken in a non-metal container. Remove skin from chicken and pierce in several places with a fork. Add chicken to marinade, making sure that all pieces are submerged. Cover and refrigerate for at least 2 hours (or preferably overnight).
2. Remove chicken from marinade and broil or barbeque for 15 to 20 minutes per side, until cooked through.

Chicken is cooked when the meat is no longer pink near the bone and the juices run clear when pierced with a sharp knife.

Secret for Success!

Makes 6 servings.
Exchanges for each serving of 1 chicken breast:
1/2 Fruit
4 Very lean meat

7g Carbohydrate, 29g Protein, 2g Fat, 160 cal
(7g available Carbohydrates)

Chicken A La King

4 halves (1 lb)	Chicken breasts, skinless, boneless
1/2 cup	Onions, chopped
2 cups	Mushrooms, sliced
1	Red peppers, diced
1	can (10oz) Chicken broth, diluted
3 tbsp	All purpose flour
2 tbsp	Sherry
1 cup	Peas, frozen
3/4 cup	'Light' sour cream

1. Lightly coat a large non-stick skillet with cooking spray and place over medium-high heat. Cut chicken into bite-size cubes and add to hot pan. Cook, stirring frequently, for 5 minutes. Add onions, mushrooms, & peppers.
2. Continue to cook, stirring occasionally, for another 8 -10 minutes, until chicken is cooked through and vegetables are tender.
3. Measure broth, sherry & flour into a jar with a tight fitting lid and shake well to blend. Stir into chicken mixture. Add frozen peas. Bring to a boil, reduce heat and simmer until bubbly and thickened.
4. Stir in sour cream and heat gently; do not allow to boil. Serve over rice, pasta or in patty shells.

This recipe freezes well so make a double batch
and freeze half for a 'busy-night' dinner.

Makes 6 servings.
Exchanges for each serving of 1/6th recipe:

1/2 Starch	3 Very lean meat
1 Vegetable	

13g Carbohydrate, 24g Protein, 3g Fat, 197 cal
(13g available Carbohydrates)

Crunchy Parmesan Chicken

1 cup	Crispy rice cereal
1/4 cup	Parmesan cheese, grated
1 tsp	Garlic powder
1 tsp	Paprika
1/2 tsp	Salt
1/2 tsp	Pepper
1/4 cup	Buttermilk, low fat
4 whole (1 lb)	Chicken legs, divided into drumsticks & thighs

1. Preheat oven to 350°F. Lightly coat a baking pan with cooking spray. With a rolling pin crush crispy rice cereal into coarse crumbs.
2. Combine cereal crumbs, parmesan cheese, garlic powder, paprika, salt, & pepper in a shallow dish (a pie plate). Pour buttermilk in a different dish.
3. Remove skin from chicken. Dip chicken pieces into the buttermilk and then roll them in the crumb mixture to coat completely.
4. Place chicken pieces on prepared baking pan, arranging the pieces so that they don't touch.
5. Bake 1 hour, until the chicken is cooked through.

time for a change

For a Mexican flavor substitute crushed tortilla chips for the cereal crumbs and taco seasoning for the garlic & paprika.

Makes 4 servings.
Exchanges for each serving of 2 pieces:
1/2 Starch   1/2 Fat
4 Very lean meat

8g Carbohydrate, 30g Protein, 7g Fat, 217 cal
(8g available Carbohydrates)

Coq Au Vin

3 slices	Bacon, diced
3 halves (3/4 lb)	Chicken breasts
3 whole (3/4 lb)	Chicken legs, divided into drumsticks & thighs
2 tsp	Olive oil
1 1/2 cups	Baby carrots
2 cloves	Garlic, minced
2 cups	Mushrooms, sliced
1/2 cup	Onions, chopped
1 cup	White wine
3/4 cup	Chicken broth (or dehydrated broth & water)
2 tbsp	Ketchup

1. Preheat oven to 350°F. Fry bacon in a large non-stick frypan over medium heat until browned and crispy. Remove with a slotted spoon. Set aside.
2. Skin chicken pieces, cut chicken breasts in half, sprinkle with salt & pepper.
3. Add olive oil to bacon drippings in pan. Add chicken and fry over medium-high heat until golden brown, about 5 minutes per side. Remove and place in a large casserole dish. Add baby carrots and cooked bacon to chicken.
4. Add garlic, onions, & mushrooms to the frypan and saute until tender. Remove with a slotted spoon and add to the chicken. Toss gently to combine.
5. Measure wine, broth, ketchup, & flour into a jar with a tight fitting lid and shake to mix. Pour into pan drippings. Cook and stir until smooth and bubbly.
6. Pour over chicken; bake, covered 45 - 50 minutes, until chicken is cooked through.

Makes 6 servings.
Exchanges for each serving of 2 chicken pieces:
1/2 Fruit   4 Lean meat
1 Vegetable

12g Carbohydrate, 30g protein, 12g fat, 309 cal
(12g available Carbohydrates)

Arroz Con Pollo

2 tsp	Olive oil
1 lb	Chicken thighs, skinless
1 tsp	Oregano, dried
1/2 tsp	Salt
1/2 tsp	Pepper
1	Onion, chopped
2 cloves	Garlic, minced
2 stalks	Celery, sliced
1	Red pepper, chopped
1 cup	White long-grain rice, uncooked
1	can (14oz) Diced tomatoes
2 cups	Chicken broth (or dehydrated broth & water)
1 cup	Peas, frozen

1. Heat olive oil in a large skillet over medium-high heat. Sprinkle chicken with salt, pepper, & oregano. Brown in hot oil for 5 minutes per side, until golden. Remove with a slotted spoon and set aside.
2. Reduce heat to medium and to same fry pan add onion, garlic, celery, & peppers. Cook 4 - 5 minutes until vegetables soften. Add rice, cook and stir for 2 minutes. Add tomatoes & broth. Bring to a boil.
3. Reduce heat and return chicken to the pan. Cover and simmer for 25 - 30 minutes, until liquid is absorbed.
4. Add frozen peas and continue cooking for 5 minutes.

Makes 4 servings.
Exchanges for each serving of 1/4th recipe:

2 1/2 Starch	3 Very lean meat
2 Vegetable	1/2 Fat

47g Carbohydrate, 29g Protein, 7g Fat, 392 cal
(47g available Carbohydrates)

Hot Chinese Chicken Salad

8 (1 1/4lb)	Chicken thighs, skinless
2 tbsp	Cornstarch
1 tbsp	Vegetable Oil
1 clove	Garlic, minced
2 cup	Mushrooms, sliced
3 stalks	Celery, sliced diagonally
6	Green onions, chopped
1	Tomato, cut in chunks
1/2 cup	Water chestnuts, sliced
3 tbsp	Soy sauce
1/2 tsp	Ginger, ground
1/2 tsp	Pepper
2 cups	Iceberg Lettuce, shredded

1. Remove bones from chicken thighs and cut meat into 1" cubes. Roll chicken cubes in cornstarch. Heat vegetable oil over high heat in a large non-stick skillet or wok.
2. Add chicken. Stir fry quickly for 4-5 minutes, until lightly browned. Reduce heat to medium-high. Add garlic, mushrooms & celery; stir-fry 2 minutes. Add green onions, tomato & water chestnuts. Sprinkle with ginger & pepper, stir in soy sauce.
3. Cover and reduce heat to low. Simmer for 5 minutes.
4. Lightly toss hot chicken mixture with lettuce and serve immediately.

Makes 4 servings.
Exchanges for each serving of 1/4th recipe:

1/2 Starch	4 Very lean meat
1 Vegetable	1 Fat

13g Carbohydrate, 30g Protein, 9g Fat, 265 cal
(13g available Carbohydrates)

Chicken and Pasta Primavera

1 tbsp	Olive Oil
4 small (3/4lb)	Chicken breasts, boneless, skinless
1/2 tsp	Salt
1/2 tsp	Pepper
1/2 cup	Onion, chopped
2 cloves	Garlic, minced
1	Red pepper, sliced in strips
1/4 lb	Mushrooms, sliced
2 cups	Zucchini, sliced
1	can (14oz) Tomatoes, diced
2 tbsp	Balsamic (or red wine) vinegar
1/4 cup	White wine
1 tsp	Italian seasoning
2 cups	Rotini (spiral macaroni)
1/4 cup	Parmesan (or Feta) Cheese, grated

1. Heat olive oil in a large non-stick fry-pan over medium high heat. Sprinkle chicken with salt & pepper and brown on both sides. Remove and set aside.
2. Reduce heat to medium. Add onion, garlic, red pepper, mushrooms, & zucchini to the same pan and saute until vegetables begin to soften, 2 - 3 mins.
3. Stir in tomatoes, vinegar, wine & Italian seasoning. Bring to a boil.
4. Add pasta, making sure that the liquid covers it. Return chicken pieces. Reduce heat, cover and cook for 15 to 25 minutes until chicken is tender and cooked through.
5. Spinkle with Parmesan (or Feta) cheese, cook for 5 minutes.

Makes 4 servings.
Exchanges for each serving of 1/4th recipe:

2 Starch	3 Lean meat
2 Vegetable	

39g Carbohydrate, 31g Protein, 8g Fat, 367 cal
(39g available Carbohydrates)

Chicken Paella

2 tsp	Olive oil
1 lb	Chicken breast, boneless, skinless, cut in 1" cubes
4 oz	Chorizo sausage, thinly sliced
1/2 cup	Onions, chopped
2 cloves	Garlic, minced
1	Red pepper, diced
1 cup	Green beans, frozen
1 1/4 cups	White long-grain rice, uncooked
1	can (14oz) Tomatoes, diced
1/2 tsp	Thyme, dried
1/4 tsp	Saffron
1/2 tsp	Pepper
2 cups	Chicken broth (or dehydrated broth & water)
4 oz	Mussels, raw
12 large	Shrimp, raw

1. Heat oil in a large, deep skillet over medium heat. Add chicken chunks and chorizo sausage slices. Cook 7-8 mins, stirring occasionally to brown all sides.
2. Remove from pan. Add onion & garlic to same pan and cook for 3 mins.
3. Add chopped peppers & rice, toss to coat, cook for 2 mins. Stir in green beans, tomatoes, spices, & chicken broth. Bring to a boil.
4. Return chicken & sausage to the pan. Reduce heat to low, cover and simmer for 25 mins. Add shrimp & mussels, simmer for 10 mins.

healthy hint...

When cooking mussels discard any that don't close when lightly tapped before cooking or that don't open after cooking

Makes 6 servings.
Exchanges for each serving of 1/6th recipe:

2 Starch	3 Lean meat
2 Vegetable	

39g Carbohydrate, 33g Protein, 11g Fat, 405cal
(39g available Carbohydrates)

Chicken Fajita Potatoes

4 medium	Baking potatoes (russet)
1/2 lb	Chicken breast, skinless, boneless, cut in strips
2 tsp	Vegetable oil
2	Green & red peppers, sliced
1/2 cup	Onions, sliced
2 tsp	Chili powder
1 tsp	Oregano, dried
1/2 tsp	Pepper
1/2 tsp	Salt
1/3 cup	Salsa
3/4 cup	'Light' Cheddar cheese, grated
1/2 cup	'Light' sour cream

1. Scrub potatoes, prick skins with a fork and bake in 400°F oven for 55 to 60 minutes, until soft.
2. Heat 1 tsp oil in a non-stick skillet over medium-high heat. Saute chicken until cooked through, 5 - 6 mins., remove and set aside.
3. Heat remaining 1 tsp oil in the same pan. Add pepper strips and onion, cook 3 - 4 mins. or until tender, remove from heat. Return chicken to pan and toss with vegetables & spices. Stir in salsa.
4. Cut a lengthwise slit in the top of each baked potato and press open. Divide chicken mixture among potatoes. Top with grated cheese. Return to oven and bake 10 mins., or until heated through.
5. Serve topped with 'light' sour cream.

Makes 4 servings.
Exchanges for each serving of 1 potato:

3 Starch	3 Very lean meat
1 Vegetable	1 Fat

51g Carbohydrate, 26g Protein, 10g Fat, 403 cal
(51g available Carbohydrates)

Chicken Salad Wraps

4	8" whole wheat tortillas
3 halves (3/4lb)	Chicken breasts, skinless, boneless, cut in strips
1/2 cup	Onions, sliced
1 clove	Garlic, minced
2 tbsp	Lime juice
1/2 tsp	Salt
1/4 tsp	Pepper
1	Tomato, diced
2 cups	Iceberg lettuce, shredded
1/2 cup	Carrots, shredded
6	Radishes, shredded
1/3 cup	'Light' Ranch dressing

1. Preheat oven to 350°F. Wrap tortillas in foil, warm in oven for 15 minutes.
2. Lightly coat a large non-stick skillet with cooking spray and heat over medium-high heat. Add chicken, onion & garlic. Stir fry for 5 -7 minutes, until chicken is cooked through. Stir in lime juice, salt & pepper.
3. Divide mixture between the warm tortillas. Top with lettuce, tomatoes, carrots, & radish. Drizzle with ranch dressing. Roll up and serve immediately

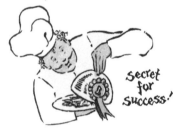

Secret for Success!

For 'brown-bagging' these wraps can be made with cold chicken but still warm the tortillas to make them more pliable for easy wrapping.

Makes 4 servings.
Exchanges for each serving of 1 wrap:

1 Starch	2 1/2 Very lean meat
2 Vegetable	1/2 Fat

26g Carbohydrate, 25g Protein, 6g Fat, 257 cal
(26g available Carbohydrates)

Popover Pizza

1 lb	Ground turkey
1/2 cup	Onions, chopped
1 clove	Garlic, minced
1	can (14oz) Tomato sauce
1 1/4 cups	Part skim Mozzarella, grated
1	Egg
2	Egg whites
1 cup	Milk, 1%
1 tbsp	Vegetable oil
1 cup	All purpose flour
1/4 tsp	Salt

1. Preheat oven to 400°F. Lightly coat a large non-stick skillet with cooking spray and heat over medium-high heat. Add ground turkey, onion & garlic. Cook and stir until meat is crumbly and no longer pink, about 5 minutes.
2. Stir in tomato sauce. Bring to a boil, reduce heat and simmer for 10 minutes.
3. Spread turkey mixture in a 9" baking dish. Sprinkle with grated mozzarella.
4. In a large mixing bowl beat the egg and egg whites until foamy. Beat in milk and oil. Combine flour and salt. Stir into egg mixture and continue beating until well blended. Pour over cheese layer.
5. Bake for 30 minutes until puffed and golden. Cut into 6 squares to serve.

Makes 6 servings of 1 square each.
Exchanges for each serving of 1 square:

1 Starch	3 Lean meat
2 Vegetable	1 Fat

25g Carbohydrate, 27g Protein, 14g Fat, 336 cal
(25 g available Carbohydrates)

Maui Meatball Kabobs

1 lb	Ground turkey
1/2 cup	Breadcrumbs
1	Egg white
1 tsp	Dijon mustard
1/2 tsp	Salt
1/4 tsp	Pepper
2/3 cup	Pineapple chunks, juice packed
1/4 cup	Soy sauce
2 tbsp	Ginger root, slivered
1 clove	Garlic, minced
4	Green onions, 1" pces
1	Green pepper, 1"cubes

1. In a medium mixing bowl combine ground turkey, breadcrumbs, egg white, mustard, salt & pepper. Mix well. Shape into 20 meatballs and place in a single layer in a non-metal dish.
2. Drain juice from pineapple into a small mixing bowl. Combine with soy sauce, ginger & garlic. Pour over meatballs. Cover and refrigerate for at least 1 hour or overnight. If using wooden skewers soak them in water for 30 mins.
3. Thread meatballs on 4 skewers alternating with pineapple, green onions, & pepper pieces. Spray with cooking oil spray.
4. Broil or grill 5-6" from heat, turning frequently to brown all sides, for 10 minutes or until meatballs are cooked through.

Makes 4 servings.
Exchanges for each serving of 1 skewer:
1 Starch
3 Lean meat

16g Carbohydrate, 24g protein, 9g fat, 252 cal
(16g available Carbohydrates)

Pesto Meatballs & Spaghetti

1 lb	Ground turkey
1/3 cup	Breadcrumbs
1/4 cup	Parmesan cheese, grated
2 tsp	Basil, dried
1/2 tsp	Garlic powder
1/2 tsp	Pepper
1/4 cup	Milk, 1%
1 tbsp	Olive oil
1/2 cup	Onions, chopped
1 1/2 cups	Mushrooms, sliced
1	Green pepper, chopped
1	can (14oz) Stewed tomatoes
1	pkg (13oz) Spaghetti

1 Combine the first seven ingredients in a large mixing bowl. Mix well and form into 24 meatballs. In a large non-stick skillet heat olive oil over medium-high heat. Add the meatballs in two batches and cook, 5 - 6 mins., until golden on all sides. Remove from pan and set aside.

2. Reduce heat to medium and in the same pan cook onions, peppers, and mushrooms for 5 mins., until softened. Return meatballs to the pan and add tomatoes. Cook 10 -15 mins.

3. Meanwhile cook spaghetti in a large pot of boiling salted water until al dente, drain. Serve meatballs and sauce over hot pasta.

chef's secret...

To ensure pasta is perfectly cooked (al dente) remove a strand from the boiling water and bite it. It should still be firm in the center.

Makes 6 servings.
Exchanges for each serving 1/6th recipe:

3 Starch   2 Lean meat
2 Vegetable

57g Carbohydrate, 26g Protein, 11g Fat, 442 cal
(57g available Carbohydrates)

Tex-Mex Turkey Burgers

1 lb	Ground turkey
1/2 cup	Corn flake crumbs
1/3 cup	Onions, chopped
2 tbsp	Jalapeno peppers, minced
1	Egg
1 clove	Garlic, minced
6	Hamburger buns
1 cup	'Light' Cheddar cheese, grated
12	Lettuce leaves
1/2 cup	Salsa
1	Avocado, sliced

1. In a large mixing bowl combine first 6 ingredients. Mix until completely blended. Shape into 6 uniform patties. Spray with vegetable oil cooking spray.
2. Heat barbeque to medium. Grill burgers 12 - 14 minutes turning once. Top with grated cheese and continue to grill 1 - 2 minutes or until cheese melts.
3. Serve on toasted buns topped with lettuce, avacado slices, and salsa.

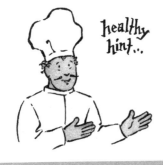

healthy hint...

Instead of eliminating foods from your diet strive for balance. For example; in this recipe using lean ground turkey for burgers allows for the option of a high fat topping like avacado.

Makes 6 servings.
Exchanges for each serving 1 burger:
2 Starch
3 Medium-fat meat

**29g Carbohydrate, 26g Protein, 18g Fat, 390 cal
(29g available Carbohydrates)**

Fish & Seafood

Lemon Shrimp & Scallop Kabobs

1/2 lb	Large raw shrimp, peeled
1/2 lb	Scallops, halved if large
2	Red, green or yellow peppers, cut into 1" cubes
4	Green onions, 1" pieces
1/4 cup	Lemon juice
1 clove	Garlic, minced
1 tbsp	Dijon mustard
1 tsp	Dill weed, dried

1. In a medium sized glass bowl combine lemon juice, garlic, dijon & dill. Add shrimp, scallops, onions, & peppers; toss gently to coat.
2. Allow to marinate in refrigerator for 30 minutes.
3. Thread seafood and vegetables alternately onto eight skewers; spray with olive oil flavored cooking spray.
4. Broil or grill over medium heat for 5-6 minutes turning once, until shrimp is pink and scallops are firm.

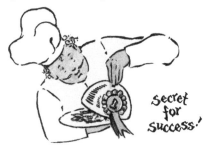

Secret for Success!

These Kabobs are especially good made with fresh seafood but frozen can be substituted. **Never** overcook shrimp and scallops or they will become tough and lose their flavor.

Make 4 servings.
Exchanges for each serving of 2 kabobs:
1 Vegetable
3 Very lean meat

5g Carbohydrate, 22g Protein, 2g Fat, 129 cal
(5g available Carbohydrates)

Grilled Halibut Burgers

1 lb	Halibut
1/2 tsp	Pepper
1/4 tsp	Salt
1 tsp	Butter
1 cup	Red onions, sliced
1 tbsp	Balsamic vinegar
1 tbsp	Splenda®
1 tsp	Thyme
2 tbsp	'Light' mayonnaise
1 tsp	Lemon juice
1 clove	Garlic, minced
8	Lettuce leaves
4	Kaiser buns

1. Divide halibut into 4 equal size servings, season with salt and pepper. Grill (or broil) 7-8 minutes, turning once, until fish is opaque and flakes easily.
2. Meanwhile melt butter in a medium non-stick skillet over medium heat. Add onions and cook 4-5 minutes, until tender. Stir in vinegar, Splenda®, & thyme; continue to cook for 1 minute.
3. Mix mayonnaise, garlic & lemon juice in a small bowl. Cut buns in half, spread with mayonnaise mixture. Place grilled fish on bun bottoms, top with onions, lettuce leaves and bun top.

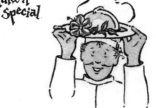

Make it Special

Vary this recipe by using different breads. Serve on crusty or Portuguese rolls, try focaccia bread, or stuff into pita pockets.

Makes 4 servings.
Exchanges for each serving of 1 burger:

2 Starch	3 Very lean meat
1 Vegetable	1/2 Fat

35g Carbohydrate, 30g Protein, 7g Fat, 338 cal
(35g available Carbohydrates)

Salmon Gremolata

1 lb	Salmon (2 fillets or 4 steaks)
1 tbsp	Olive oil
1 tbsp	Lemon juice
1 clove	Garlic, minced
1 tsp	Salt
1 tsp	Pepper
3 tbsp	Parsley, snipped
3 tbsp	Chives, snipped
1 tbsp	Lemon zest

1. Position rack about 5 - 6" from heat, preheat broiler.
2. In a small bowl combine oil, lemon juice, salt, pepper, & garlic. Brush salmon with mixture and place on a rack set in broiler pan.
3. Broil 4 - 5 minutes per side, until fish flakes easily when tested with a fork.
4. Meanwhile combine parsley, chives, & lemon zest. Top salmon with parsley mixture and serve.

chef's secret...

To make lemon zest: Wash lemon with soapy water to remove any pesticide residue and then using a grater or zester remove the outer yellow skin the 'zest'. Freeze in a freezer bag and use as needed.

Makes 4 servings.
Exchanges for each serving of 1/4th recipe:
4 Lean meat
1/2 Fat

1g Carbohydrate, 27g protein, 14g fat, 245 cal
(1g available Carbohydrates)

Salmon With Lemony Mayo

1	Onion, sliced
2	Limes, sliced
4 (3.5oz ea)	Salmon steaks
1/4 cup	Italian dressing, reduced fat
1/4 cup	Parsley, chopped
1/4 cup	'Light' mayonnaise
1 tbsp	Lemon juice
1 tsp	Lemon zest (see tip on pg. 82)
2 tbsp	Chives, snipped
1 clove	Garlic, minced

1. Lightly coat a non-metal baking dish with cooking spray.
2. Arrange half of the onion and lime slices in a single layer in the prepared baking dish. Top with salmon steaks.
3. Sprinkle half of the Italian dressing over the fish, turn and sprinkle the other side with the rest of the dressing. Top with the remaining onion and lime slices. Sprinkle with parsley. Cover and refrigerate 2 to 4 hours.
4. To make lemon mayo: mix mayonnaise, lemon juice, lemon zest, chives, & garlic in a small bowl, set aside.
5. Preheat oven to 375°F. Uncover salmon and bake 20 - 25 minutes, until fish flakes easily when tested with a fork.
6. Remove onions and limes. Top with a dollop of lemon mayonnaise & serve.

Makes 4 servings.
Each serving of 1 salmon steak:

1/2 Starch   1/2 Fat
3 Lean meat

7g Carbohydrate, 22g Protein, 12g Fat, 230 cal
(7g available Carbohydrates)

Crispy Herbed Sole

1 lb	Sole fillets, cut in serving size pieces
1/3 cup	Breadcrumbs
1/4 cup	Parmesan cheese, grated
2 tsp	Lemon juice
2 tsp	Olive oil
1 tsp	Basil, dried
1/2 tsp	Oregano, dried
1/2 tsp	Salt
1/2 tsp	Pepper

1. Preheat oven to 375°F. Lightly coat a baking sheet with cooking spray and arrange fillets in a single layer on the sheet.
2. In a small bowl toss together all the rest of the ingredients.
3. Sprinkle the fillets with the bread crumb mixture. Pat coating down lightly with your hand.
4. Bake fillets for 10-15 minutes or until fish flakes easily with a fork.

chef's secret...

Fish is easily overcooked making it dry and tasteless. Cook it just until it flakes easily when tested with a fork.

Makes 4 servings.
Exchanges for each serving of 1/4th recipe:

1/2 Starch	1/2 Fat
3 1/2 Very lean meat	

7g Carbohydrate, 26g Protein, 6g Fat, 190 cal
(7g available Carbohydrates)

Pepper Sole Veronique

2 tbsp	All purpose flour
1/2 tsp	Thyme, dried
1/4 tsp	Salt
1/4 tsp	Pepper
1 lb	Sole fillets, cut in serving size pieces
1 tbsp	Butter
1	Red pepper, julienne strips
3 tbsp	Green onions, finely chopped
3/4 cup	Green grapes, halved
2 tbsp	White wine
1/4 cup	Slivered almonds, toasted

1. Preheat oven to 300°F. Spread almonds on a cookie sheet and toast in preheated oven for 5 -10 mins, until golden. Set aside.
2.Combine flour, thyme, salt & pepper in a shallow dish. Coat sole fillets in flour mixture.
3. Melt butter in a large skillet over medium heat. Fry coated fillets in melted butter for 3 minutes per side or until fish flakes easily when tested with a fork. Transfer to a serving dish and keep warm in preheated oven.
3. Add red pepper strips to same frypan and saute for 3 minutes. Add green onion and continue to cook for 1 min, add grapes & wine. Cook until heated through, about 2 minutes.
4. Spoon pepper/ grape mixture over fish and sprinkle with toasted almonds.

Makes 4 servings.
Exchanges for each serving of 1/4th recipe:
1/2 Fruit
3 Lean meat

8g Carbohydrate, 23g protein, 6g fat, 188 cal
(8g available Carbohydrates)

Fresh Salsa Snapper

1 lb	Red Snapper fillets
2	Roma tomatoes, chopped
1	Green pepper, chopped
1	Jalapeno pepper, minced
3	Green onions, chopped
3 tbsp	Cilantro, snipped
1/4 tsp	Salt
1/4 cup	White wine

1. Preheat oven to 300°F. Lightly coat a large non-stick skillet with cooking spray. Heat over medium heat.
2. Cut fish into serving size portions and arrange in a single layer in skillet. Cook for 3 minutes. Turn and continue cooking for 3 - 4 minutes, until fish flakes easily when tested with a fork. Remove and keep warm in oven.
3. Add tomato, peppers & onion to the pan. Cook over medium heat stirring frequently for 3 - 4 minutes, until pepper is tender. Stir in salt, cilantro, & wine, heat through.
4. Spoon hot salsa over fish and serve immediately.

For moist, flavorful fish check often for doneness. Also, use caution when using hot peppers, even the fumes can sting!

Secret for Success!

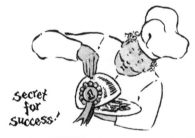

Makes 4 servings.
Exchanges for each serving of 1/4th recipe:
1/2 Vegetable
3 1/2 Very lean meat

3g Carbohydrate, 24g Protein, 2g Fat, 148 cal
(3g available Carbohydrates)

Baked Fish Picante

1 cup	Mushrooms, sliced
1	Green or red pepper, sliced
1/4 cup	Onions, sliced
1 lb	Snapper or Flounder fillets
1 tsp	Oregano, dried
1/2 tsp	Salt
1/4 tsp	Pepper
1/2 cup	Salsa
1 cup	Monterey Jack cheese, grated

1. Preheat oven to 450°F. Place mushrooms, peppers & onions in a microwave-safe cooking dish. Cover with plastic wrap and cook 2-3 minutes, until barely tender.
2. Lightly coat a 9" baking dish with cooking spray. Arrange fish fillets in a single layer, folding thin ends under.
3. Sprinkle with oregano, salt, & pepper. Spoon cooked vegetables over fish, top with salsa.
4. Bake for 10 minutes. Sprinkle with cheese and bake for 3-4 minutes more until cheese has melted and fish flakes easily when tested with a fork.

Makes 4 servings.
Exchanges for each serving of 1/4th recipe:
1 Vegetable
4 Lean meat

6g Carbohydrate, 30g Protein, 10g Fat, 230cal
(6g available Carbohydrates)

Fish & Chips with Tartar Sauce

Tartar Sauce

1/2 cup	Plain Yogurt, low fat
1/4 cup	Pickles, finely chopped
1/4 cup	Celery, finely chopped
2 tbsp	Green onions, finely chopped
1 clove	Garlic, minced

Fish & Chips

1 1/2 lb	Baking potatoes (5 medium)
1 1/2 tbsp	Olive oil
1 tbsp	Paprika
2	Egg whites
1/4 cup	Cornmeal
1/4 cup	Breadcrumbs, dry
1/4 cup	All purpose flour
1 lb	Cod, Flounder, or Halibut, in serving-size pieces

1. To make tartar sauce: mix first five ingredients together and set aside.
2. Preheat oven to 450°F. Spray a baking sheet with cooking spray.
3. Scrub potatoes & cut into long thin wedges. Soak in cold salted water for 10 to15 mins. Drain, pat dry, & spread in single layer on baking sheet. Spray with cooking spray. Sprinkle with salt and 1 tsp paprika. Bake for 20 -25 minutes.
4. In a flat dish beat egg whites with a fork. In a separate dish combine cornmeal, breadcrumbs, remaining paprika, salt & pepper. Place flour in a separate dish. Dip fish into flour, then egg whites, then cornmeal mixture.
5. Heat the olive oil in a large skillet over medium high heat. Fry fish 3 - 4 minutes per side or until cooked through. Serve with tartar sauce & 'fries'.

Makes 5 servings.
Exchanges for each serving of 1/5 recipe:
2 1/2 Starch
3 Very lean meat

39g Carbohydrate, 25g protein, 5g fat, 315 cal
(39g available Carbohydrates)

Cod Crumble

1 lb	Cod fillets
1	can (10 3/4oz) Cream of mushroom soup, '98% fat free'
2 tbsp	White wine
1/2 cup	'Light' Cheddar cheese, grated
5	Green onions, chopped
3 slices	Bacon, cooked & crumbled

1. Preheat oven to 350°F.
2. Cut cod into serving size portions Arrange in a single layer in a baking dish.
3. In a small bowl combine the soup and wine. Pour over fish. Sprinkle cheese, green onions & crumbled bacon on top.
4. Bake uncovered for 30 mins, until fish flakes easily when tested with a fork.

Makes 4 servings.
Exchanges for each serving of 1/4th recipe:
1/2 Starch   1 Fat
3 1/2 Very lean meat

7g Carbohydrate, 27g Protein, 8g Fat, 172 cal
(7g available Carbohydrates)

Fish Substitution Chart

If your recipe calls for:

Sole	Red Snapper	Cod	Tuna
Substitute:			
Flounder, Fluke, Trout	Rockfish, Orange Roughy, Grouper	Haddock, Halibut	Swordfish, Salmon
Characteristics:			
Thin, tender, lean, mild	Thin, firm, lean, mild-medium	Thick, firm, lean, mild	Thick, firm, slightly oily

Mexi Cod with Pasta Shells

1 1/2 cups	Medium pasta shells
2 tsp	Olive oil
1/2 cup	Onions, chopped
1	can (14oz) Tomatoes, diced
1 tbsp	Chili powder
1/2 tsp	Cumin
1 tsp	Oregano, dried
1/2 tsp	Pepper
1 tsp	Salt
1	Green pepper, cut in strips
1 lb	Cod fillets
3/4 cup	'Light' Cheddar cheese, grated

1. Cook pasta shells according to package directions, drain and set aside.
2. Heat olive oil in a medium-sized saucepan over medium-high heat. Add onion and cook until tender, about 4 minutes.
3. Add tomatoes, seasonings, & green pepper strips. Bring to a boil, reduce heat and simmer for 5 minutes. Stir in cooked pasta shells.
4. Preheat oven to 350°F. Lightly coat a 9" baking dish with cooking spray. Spoon pasta mixture into dish.
5. Cut fish into serving size pieces. Nestle fish in pasta, folding thin ends under as necessary to fit in dish. Spoon some sauce over fish.
6. Bake covered for 30 minutes. Uncover, sprinkle with cheese and bake 5 minutes longer.

Makes 4 servings.
Exchanges for each serving of 1/4th recipe:
2 Starch   3 Lean meat
2 Vegetable

40g Carbohydrate, 33g Protein, 9g Fat, 378 cal
(40g available Carbohydrates)

Tuna Tetrazzini

1	pkg (13oz) Spaghetti
1	can (10 3/4oz) Cream of mushroom soup, '98% fat free'
1 cup	'Light' Cheddar cheese, grated
1/2 cup	Milk, 1%
1/4 cup	White wine
1/2 tsp	Oregano, dried
1/2 tsp	Pepper
1/2 tsp	Salt
2	cans (6oz) Tuna, drained
1	pkg (10oz) frozen Spinach, thawed & squeezed dry
1/4 cup	Parmesan cheese, grated

1. Cook pasta according to instructions on the package, drain and set aside.
2. Preheat oven to 350°F. Lightly coat a 9 x 13" baking dish with non-stick cooking spray.
3. In a mixing bowl combine the mushroom soup, cheddar cheese, milk, wine, oregano, salt & pepper. Add well-drained tuna, spinach & cooked pasta. Toss gently to combine.
4. Spoon into prepared baking dish. Sprinkle with parmesan cheese.
5. Bake uncovered for 25 - 30 minutes, until bubbly & lightly browned.

Makes 6 servings.
Exchanges for each serving of 1/6th recipe:
3 Starch   3 1/2 Very lean meat
1 Vegetable   1/2 Fat

50g Carbohydrate, 35g Protein, 8g Fat, 413 cal
(50g available Carbohydrates)

Deep Dish Tuna Pie

1 crust	Betty Crocker® piecrust mix
1/2 cup	Onions, chopped
1	can (10 3/4oz) Cream of mushroom soup, '98% fat free'
1/3 cup	Milk, 1%
1/4 cup	Parmesan cheese, grated
2 tbsp	White wine
1 tsp	Dill weed, dried
1/2 tsp	Pepper
1 1/2 cups	Peas & carrots, frozen
2 cups	Broccoli, cut in small florets
3	cans (6oz)Tuna, drained

1. Prepare pie crust according to package instructions but don't roll out. Cover and set aside.
2. Spray a large non-stick frypan with cooking spray. Add onion, cook over medium heat until soft and translucent, 4-5 mins.
3. Stir in soup, milk, parmesan cheese, wine, dill and pepper. Cook and stir until bubbly. Stir in vegetables and heat through. Break tuna into chunks and gently stir in. Spoon into a 2qt round casserole dish.
4. On a lightly floured surface roll out pastry until slightly bigger then the top of the casserole. Carefully place the pastry over the casserole and flute edges. Poke the pastry all over with fork to vent.
5. Bake at 400°F for 40-45 minutes. Cut into 6 wedges to serve.

Makes 6 servings.
Exchanges for each serving of 1 wedge:
1 Starch
1 Vegetable   3 1/2 Lean meat

21g Carbohydrate, 29g Protein, 12g Fat, 326 cal
(21g available Carbohydrates)

Salmon And Rice Casserole

2 cups	Mushrooms, sliced
1	Red pepper, chopped
5oz (1/2pkg)	Frozen chopped Spinach, thawed & drained
1	can (10 3/4oz) Cream of mushroom soup, '98% fat free'
1/2 cup	Milk, 1%
1 1/2 cups	'Light' Cheddar cheese, grated
3 cups	Cooked white rice
2	cans (7.5oz) Salmon
1/2 cup	Breadcrumbs

1. Preheat oven to 350°F. Lightly coat a 2 qt casserole dish with cooking spray. Put mushrooms in microwave-safe dish, cover with plastic wrap, & microcook until tender, 3-4 minutes. Mix with red pepper & spinach.
2. In a medium saucepan heat soup, milk, & 1 cup grated cheese over medium heat until the cheese melts.
3. Spread 1/3 of the cooked rice in the prepared casserole dish. Layer with 1/2 of the salmon, and 1/2 of the mushroom mixture. Repeat layers. Top with remaining 1/3 of the rice. Pour soup mixture over all.
4. Combine remaining 1/2 cup grated cheese and breadcrumbs. Sprinkle over casserole. Bake for 30 minutes.

chef's secret...

Thawed frozen spinach holds a lot of water even when drained in a colander. Wring it out with your hands to remove the excess.

Makes 6 servings.
Exchanges for each serving of 1/6th recipe:

2 Starch	2 1/2 Lean meat
1 1/2 Vegetable	1/2 Fat

36g Carbohydrate, 26g Protein, 13g Fat, 365 cal
(36g available Carbohydrates)

Salmon Strudel

1	pkg (10oz) Spinach, thawed
1 cup	Zucchini, shredded
2	cans (7.5oz) Sockeye salmon, drained
4 oz	'Light' cream cheese
3/4 cup	Cottage cheese, 1%
2	Eggs
1/2 tsp	Dill weed, dried
1/2 tsp	Salt
10 sheets	Phyllo pastry
1 tbsp	Breadcrumbs, dry
1 tbsp	Butter, melted

1. Preheat oven to 350°F. Drain spinach well and squeeze out excess moisture. Pat zucchini dry with paper towels. Combine spinach, zucchini, salmon, cream cheese, cottage cheese, eggs, dill, & salt. Set aside.
2. Place two sheets of phyllo, one on top of the other, on a piece of waxed paper on a work space. Spray with butter flavored cooking spray and sprinkle with 1 tsp of breadcrumbs. Continue layering three more times, ending with 2 phyllo sheets.
3. Spoon on the salmon mixture, covering half of the phyllo lengthwise and leaving a 1" border. Starting with the salmon covered half, roll up, tucking in the ends. Place the roll, seam side down on a baking sheet and brush the top with the melted butter. Cut 12 slashes in the top.
4. Bake 35-40 mins until golden. Let sit for 5 mins, then slice into 6 pieces.

Makes 6 servings.
Exchanges for each serving of 1 slice:
2 Starch
3 Medium-fat meat

30g Carbohydrate, 26g protein, 15g fat, 371cal
(30g available Carbohydrates)

Beef & Pork

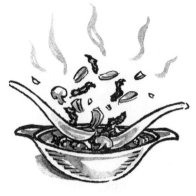

	Page

Burgundy Beef Stew

1 tbsp	Vegetable oil
1 lb	Lean stewing beef, cut in 1 1/2" cubes
1 cup	Onions, sliced
2 cloves	Garlic, minced
2 cups	Beef broth, canned, 'ready to use'
1/4 cup	Tomato sauce
5	Carrots, sliced
2 cups	Mushrooms, quartered
4	Potatoes, peeled & cut in cubes
3 stalks	Celery, sliced
2 tbsp	Cornstarch
1/4 cup	Red Burgundy wine

1. Heat oil in a large heavy saucepan over medium-high heat. Add beef cubes and saute for 5-6 minutes, until brown on all sides. Add onions and garlic and continue to cook for 2 minutes.

2. Stir in beef broth, tomato sauce and just enough water to cover; bring to a boil. Reduce heat to simmer, cover and simmer for 1 1/2 to 2 hours.

3. Add carrots, mushrooms, potatoes, & celery. Cover and continue to simmer for 30 minutes.

4. In a small bowl whisk the red wine into the cornstarch; stir into stew. Increase heat to medium-high and cook until gravy is thickened and bubbly. Cook, uncovered, for 2-3 minutes.

Makes 6 servings.
Exchanges for each serving of 1/6th recipe:

2 1/2 Starch	2 1/2 Lean meat
1 Vegetable	

27g Carbohydrate, 23g Protein, 7g Fat, 283 cal
(27g available Carbohydrates)

Beef Stroganoff

1 tsp	Vegetable oil
1 lb	Sirloin steak, cut in thin strips
1/2 cup	Onions, chopped
2 cloves	Garlic, minced
1 1/2 cups	Mushrooms, sliced
2 tbsp	All purpose flour
1 cup	Beef broth, canned, 'ready to use'
3 tbsp	Red wine
2 tsp	Dijon mustard
1/2 tsp	Salt
1/2 tsp	Pepper
2/3 cup	'Light' sour cream
1/4 cup	Parsley, chopped

1. In a large non-stick skillet heat vegetable oil over medium-high heat. When hot, add beef strips and saute until browned on all sides, about 5 minutes. Remove from pan.
2. Reduce heat to medium, add onions & garlic, cook for 2 minutes. Add mushrooms and continue cooking 5-6 minutes, until mushrooms are tender.
3. Whisk flour into the wine to make a paste. Stir beef broth, wine/flour mixture, mustard, salt & pepper into the pan. Return beef to pan, cook and stir 5 minutes. Stir in sour cream. Heat through but don't allow to boil.
4. Sprinkle with parsley and serve immediately over hot noodles or rice*.

Makes 4 servings.
Exchanges for each serving of 1/4th recipe:
2 Vegetables
3 1/2 Lean meat
*Exchanges do not include rice or noodles

10g Carbohydrate, 28g Protein, 8g Fat, 253 cal
(10g available Carbohydrates)

Peppered Roast Beef

2 1/4 lb	Eye of round roast
2 tsp	Olive oil
2 tbsp	Dijon mustard
2 cloves	Garlic, minced
1 tsp	Oregano, dried
1 tbsp	Black peppercorns, cracked
2 tsp	Coarse (pickling) salt

1. Preheat oven to 325°F.
2. Combine olive oil, mustard, garlic & oregano. Rub over roast. Sprinkle all sides with freshly cracked pepper and coarse salt. Place on a rack in a shallow roasting pan.
3. Cook about 1 hour or until meat is medium rare and registers 140°F on a meat thermometer.
4. Let stand for 20 minutes before slicing. Serve with mushroom gravy (pg 99).

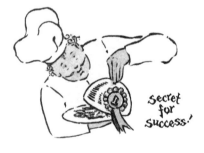

Secret
for
Success!

Never carve a roast until you've let it rest for 20 minutes. During cooking the juices retreat away from the heat source and into the center of the roast. As the roast stands the juices redistribute themselves throughout the meat.

Makes 8 servings.
Exchanges for each serving of 2 slices:
4 Lean meat

1g Carbohydrate, 27g Protein, 12g Fat, 232 cal
(1g available Carbohydrate)

Mushroom Gravy

1 tsp	Vegetable oil
1 cup	Mushrooms, diced
1 1/2 cups	Beef broth, canned 'ready to use'
1/2 tsp	Thyme, dried
1/2 tsp	Onion powder
1/2 tsp	Garlic powder
1/2 tsp	Pepper
3 tbsp	Red wine
2 tbsp	Cornstarch

1. Heat the oil in a medium sized saucepan over medium-low heat. Add mushrooms and saute until they have given up their liquid and are soft, about 4 minutes.
2. Add the broth and spices. Boil gently for 5 minutes.
3. Stir together the wine and the cornstarch to make a smooth paste. Whisk into broth mixture. Simmer and stir until smooth and thickened.

chef's secret...

Gravy too thin? Keep cooking to evaporate some moisture OR mix 2 tsp cornstarch in a 1/4 cup cold water, add to gravy, cook until desired thickness.

Makes 8 servings.
Exchanges for each serving of 1/4 cup:
1/2 Vegetable

3g Carbohydrate, 1g Protein, 1g Fat, 23 cal
(3g available Carbohydrates)

Fast & Healthy Stir Fry

1/4 cup	Soy sauce
1 tbsp	Cornstarch
1 tbsp	Splenda®
1 tsp	Chili powder
1 lb	Sirloin tip steak, cut in strips
1 tbsp	Vegetable oil
1 clove	Garlic, minced
1 tbsp	Ginger, slivered
2 stalks	Celery, diagonally sliced
3	Carrots, diagonally sliced
2 cups	Broccoli, chopped
2 cups	Mushrooms, sliced
1	Red pepper, chopped
4	Green onions, sliced

1. Stir first four ingredients together with 1/2 cup of water to make a sauce, set aside. Cut all vegetables and set aside.
2. Heat vegetable oil in a large non-stick skillet or wok over high heat. Add mea garlic, and ginger. Stir-fry for 3 minutes or until lightly browned.
4. Add vegetables to the wok and stir-fry for 2 minutes. Drizzle with sauce. Cover and cook 5 minutes, until the vegetables are tender crisp.

Stir-frys are quick and easy if you prepare all of the ingredients first. This recipe can be varied by using chicken, pork, or prawns instead of steak, and any variety of seasonal vegetables.

Secret for Success!

Makes 6 servings.
Exchanges for each serving of 1/6th recipe:
2 Vegetable
2 1/2 Lean meat

10g Carbohydrate, 21g Protein, 6g Fat, 175 cal
(8g available Carbohydrates)

Pepper Steak

1 lb	Sirloin steak
1 tbsp	Paprika
1 tbsp	Olive oil
2 cloves	Garlic, minced
1 1/2 cups	Beef broth
4	Green onions, chopped
2	Green peppers, cut in strips
1 tbsp	Cornstarch
2 tbsp	Soy sauce
3	Fresh tomatoes, cut in wedges

1. Cut the steak into thin strips. Sprinkle with paprika.
2. Heat olive oil in a large skillet over medium-high heat. Add beef strips and garlic, saute about 4 minutes, until meat is brown. Add broth, cover and simmer for 20 minutes.
3. Add onions & green peppers. Cover and cook 5 minutes more.
4. In a small bowl blend 1/4 cup water, soy sauce, & cornstarch. Stir into meat mixture. Cook and stir until clear and thickened, about 2 minutes.
5. Gently stir in tomatoes and continue cooking just until heated through. Serve over hot rice.

chef's secret...

It is easier to slice raw steak into thin strips if you partially freeze it first for 30 minutes; until it is firm.

Makes 6 servings.
Exchanges for each serving of 1/6th recipe:
1 Vegetable
2 1/2 Lean meat

7g Carbohydrate, 19g Protein, 6g Fat, 162 cal
(7g available Carbohydrates)

Beef & Mac Casserole

1 lb	Lean ground beef
2 cups	Mushrooms, sliced
1/2 cup	Onions, chopped
1 clove	Garlic, minced
1/2 tsp	Basil, dried
1/2 tsp	Oregano, dried
1/2 tsp	Chili powder
1/2 tsp	Pepper
1/4 tsp	Salt
1	can (5oz) Tomato paste
1	can (14oz) Tomatoes, diced
6 cups	Elbow macaroni, cooked
1 1/2 cups	Cottage cheese (1%)
1 cup	Part skim Mozzarella cheese, grated

1. In a large non-stick skillet cook ground beef over medium heat until brown & crumbly. Add mushrooms, onions, & garlic. Continue to cook until mushrooms are soft and onion is translucent, about 4 minutes.
2. Stir in spices, tomato paste & tomatoes; simmer for 10 minutes.
3. Remove from heat, add cooked macaroni. Toss gently to combine.
4. Spoon half of the macaroni/meat mixture into a 13 x 9" casserole dish. Spread with cottage cheese and then the remaining macaroni mixture.
5. Cover and bake for 25 minutes. Uncover, sprinkle with grated mozzarella, and bake uncovered for 10 minutes.

Makes 8 servings.
Exchanges for each serving of 1/8th recipe:
2 1/2 Starch   1/2 Fat
3 Lean meat

38g Carbohydrate, 29g Protein, 13g fat, 397 cal
(38g available Carbohydrates)

Spicy Joes

3/4 lb	Lean ground beef
1/4 cup	Green peppers, chopped
1/4 cup	Onions, diced
1 clove	Garlic, minced
1	can (14oz) Kidney beans, drained & rinsed
1 tsp	Salt
1/2 tsp	Pepper
1/2 cup	Corn, frozen
1	can (14oz)Tomatoes with green chilies
1/4 tsp	Tabasco sauce
4	Hamburger buns

1. In a large skillet, over medium-high heat, saute beef, peppers, onion, & garlic, stirring often. Cook until meat is browned & crumbly, about 6-7 minutes. Drain fat.
2. Mash kidney beans slightly with a fork. Stir into ground beef mixture along with tomatoes, corn, salt & pepper, tabasco and 1/4 cup of water. Simmer 5-10 minutes, stirring occasionally, until heated through.
3. Cut buns, place cut side up on a baking sheet; toast under broiler.
4. Spoon beef mixture onto open-faced toasted buns and serve.

Makes 4 servings.
Exchanges for each serving of 2 bun halves:
2 1/2 Starch   2 1/2 Medium-fat meat
1 Vegetable

42g Carbohydrate, 27g Protein, 16g Fat, 451 cal
(42g available Carbohydrates)

Barbequed Pork Fajitas

4	8" Whole wheat tortillas
1 tsp	Chili powder
1 tsp	Cumin, ground
1/2 tsp	Garlic powder
1/4 tsp	Cayenne pepper
3/4 lb	Pork loin, cut in thin strips
1/2 cup	Red onion, sliced
1	Green pepper, cut in strips
1	Red pepper, cut in strips
2 tbsp	Barbecue sauce
2 tbsp	Salsa
1/2 tsp	Tabasco sauce

1. Preheat oven to 350°F. Wrap tortillas in foil, place in oven for 15 minutes.
2. Combine spices in a plastic bag. Add pork strips; shake to coat with spices.
3. Spray a large non-stick frypan with cooking spray and heat over medium-high heat. When the pan is hot, add the pork and saute for 2 minutes.
4. Add the onion and pepper. Continue to saute for 3-4 minutes, until pork is no longer pink and vegetables are tender crisp.
5. Stir in barbecue sauce, salsa & tabasco. Heat through for 3 minutes.
6. Spoon 1/4 of the mixture in the center of each tortilla, roll up and serve.

Makes 4 servings.
Exchanges for each serving of 1 fajita:

1 Starch	3 Very lean meat
1/2 Fruit	1/2 Fat

23g Carbohydrate, 24g Protein, 7g Fat, 244 cal
(23g available Carbohydrates)

Asian Pork Kabobs

1/4 cup	Soy sauce
2 tbsp	'Reduced fat' Peanut butter
2 tbsp	Rice vinegar
1 tbsp	Lemon juice
2 tsp	Worcestershire sauce
1 tsp	Hot dry mustard
2 tbsp	Cilantro, chopped
3/4 lb	Pork tenderloin

1. Mix first 7 ingredients in a small bowl and then transfer to a sealable food storage bag.
2. Cut the pork into 1 1/2" cubes and add to the marinade in the bag. Refrigerate for at least 1 hour, turning frequently.
3. Preheat broiler and position oven rack 5 - 6" from the element. Spray broiler pan with cooking spray. Thread pork onto 4 metal skewers.
4. Broil kabobs 4 - 5 minutes. Turn, baste with marinade and continue broiling 4-5 minutes until lightly browned on both sides.

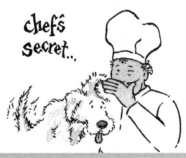

chef's secret...

These kabobs can be barbecued. If you use bamboo skewers soak them in water for 30 minutes first so they won't burn.

Makes 4 servings.
Exchanges for each serving of 1 kabob:
1 Vegetable   1 Fat
3 Very lean meat

5g Carbohydrate, 22g Protein, 6g Fat, 169 cal
(5g available Carbohydrates)

Ham & Pineapple Kabobs

1	can (14oz) Pineapple chunks, juice packed
3 tbsp	Orange juice
1 tbsp	Parsley, dried
1/2 tsp	Garlic powder
1/2 tsp	Tabasco sauce
1 tbsp	Olive oil
1 1/4lb	Cooked ham, cut in 1 1/2" cubes
2	Green peppers, cut in 1 1/2" cubes
6	Green onions, cut in 1" pcs

1. Drain pineapple and save the juice. Combine 2 Tbsp pineapple juice, orange juice, parsley, garlic powder, tabasco sauce, & olive oil in a small bowl.
2. Thread cubes of ham, pineapple, peppers, & green onions alternately onto 6 long metal skewers. Brush all sides with juice mixture.
3. Place skewers on preheated barbeque. Grill, turning once and basting with juice mixture. Cook until vegetables are softened, about 10 minutes.

time for a change

Make these versatile kabobs with chicken or pork tenderloin, or with prawns & scallops. Adjust cooking time to ensure the meat is cooked through. Prawns & scallops are quickest; just cook until prawns turn pink. They also can be broiled instead of barbecued.

Makes 6 servings.
Exchanges for each serving of one kabob:
1 Fruit
3 Lean meat

14g Carbohydrate, 22g Protein, 8g Fat, 220 cal
(14g available Carbohydrates)

Oven Barbecued Pork Chops

1 1/4lbs (6 small)	Pork loin chops
1/3 cup	Ketchup
1/4 cup	Cider vinegar
1 clove	Garlic, minced
1 tbsp	Splenda®
2 tsp	Worcestershire sauce
1/4 tsp	Tabasco sauce
1/2 cup	Onions, chopped
2	Green or red peppers, sliced

1. Trim fat from pork chops. Place in a single layer in a 9 x 13" non-metal baking dish. In a small bowl combine ketchup, vinegar, garlic, Splenda®, worcestershire sauce, & tabasco. Pour over chops and marinate in refrigerator for 1 hour or more.
2. Preheat oven to 350°F.
3. Sprinkle pork chops with onions and peppers, cover with foil and bake for 30 minutes.
4. Uncover, turn chops over. Continue baking, uncovered, for 20 minutes.

Makes 6 servings.
Exchanges for each serving of one pork chop:
1/2 Fruit   1/2 Fat
3 Very lean meat

7g Carbohydrate, 20g Protein, 6g Fat, 165 cal
(7g available Carbohydrates)

Teriyaki Pork Chops

1 lb (4 medium)	Pork loin chops
1/2 tsp	Ginger, ground
1/2 tsp	Garlic powder
1	Red pepper, thinly sliced
2	Carrot, shredded
4	Green onions, chopped
1/4 cup	Orange juice
1/4 cup	Teriyaki sauce
2 tsp	Cornstarch
1/4 tsp	Tabasco sauce

1. Trim fat from pork chops. Sprinkle both sides with ginger & garlic. Preheat a heavy non-stick skillet over medium-high heat. Add pork chops and cook 10 to 15 minutes turning once, until browned outside & cooked through. Remove from pan and keep warm.

2. Add red pepper, shredded carrot & green onion to same pan. Stir-fry over medium heat 2-3 minutes or until tender crisp.

3. In a small bowl combine orange juice, teriyaki sauce, cornstarch & tabasco sauce; add to vegetables. Cook and stir until thickened and bubbly. Spoon over pork chops to serve.

Makes 4 servings.
Exchanges for each serving of 1 pork chop:
2 Vegetable
2 1/2 Lean meat

10g Carbohydrate, 21g Protein, 6g Fat, 183 cal
(10g available Carbohydrates)

Meatless Main Dishes

Pizza Pockets

1 envelope	Yeast, 'rapid rise'
2 tsp	Vegetable Oil
1/4 tsp	Salt
1 1/2 cups	All purpose flour
2 cups	Broccoli florets
2 cups	Mushrooms, sliced
1/2 cup	Onions, chopped
1	Green pepper, chopped
1/2 cup	Tomato sauce
1 tsp	Oregano
1 tsp	Garlic powder
1 1/2 cups	Part skim Mozzarella cheese, grated

1. In a medium mixing bowl combine yeast with 1/2 cup very warm tap water. Stir until dissolved. Add oil and salt. Stir in flour until mixture forms a soft dough. Turn onto a lightly floured surface and knead for 5 minutes.
2. Form dough into a ball. Coat with cooking spray and let sit 15 -20 minutes.
3. Preheat oven to 425°F. Sprinkle a baking sheet with cornmeal.
4. Cook vegetables in microwave for 3 - 4 minutes, until tender crisp. Rinse in cold water and let drain. Mix with tomato sauce, oregano, & garlic.
5. Divide pizza dough into 4 balls. On lightly floured surface roll each ball into a 8" circle. Divide vegetable mixture onto each round, covering half and leaving a 1 1/2" border. Sprinkle with mozzarella.
6. Fold dough over filling. Turn edges up and over, pressing firmly to seal.
7. Place on baking sheet. Slit tops to vent. Bake 20 minutes, or until golden.

Makes 4 servings.
Exchanges for each serving of 1 pizza pocket:
3 Starch   1 1/2 Medium-fat Meat
1 Vegetable

46g Carboyhdrate, 21g protein, 11g Fat, 381 cal
(46g available Carboydrates)

Unstuffed Cabbage Rolls

1 1/4 cups	Brown rice, raw
4 cups	Cabbage, coarsely shredded
1/2 cup	Onion, chopped
1	can (28oz) Stewed tomatoes
2 tbsp	Lemon juice
1 tbsp	Brown sugar
1 tsp	Dill weed, dried
1/2 tsp	Allspice, ground
1 tsp	Salt
1/2 tsp	Pepper
12 oz	Morningstar Farms® 'Burger Style Recipe Crumbs'

1. Cook rice in 2 1/2 cups salted water for 40 minutes.
2. While rice is cooking, lightly coat a large non-stick skillet with cooking spray. Preheat over medium-high heat. Add cabbage & onions. Cook 5 - 6 mins., until cabbage is wilted and beginning to brown.
3. Add remaining ingredients, except ground round; bring to a boil. Reduce heat and simmer for 15 minutes.
4. Add veggie ground round, stirring to crumble. Heat through for 5 minutes.
5. Serve with hot rice.

'Burger Style Recipe Crumbs' is a precooked soy protein product. For best results it should be added in the last few minutes of cooking.

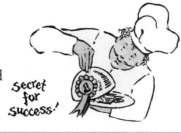

Secret for Success!

Makes 6 servings.
Exchanges for each serving of 1/6th recipe:

2 Starch	1 Vegetable
1 Other Carbohydrate	1 1/2 Very Lean Meat

51g Carbohydrate, 19g protein, 2g Fat, 285 cal
(51g available Carbohydrates)

Sloppy Jills

1/2 cup	Onions, diced
1 clove	Garlic, minced
1	Green pepper, diced
1/2 cup	Carrots, grated
1	can (14oz) Kidney beans, drained & rinsed
1	can (14oz) Stewed tomatoes
1/2 cup	Corn, frozen kernels
1 tbsp	Cider vinegar
1 tbsp	Splenda®
1/2 tsp	Salt
4	Hamburger buns
1/2 cup	'Light' Cheddar cheese, grated

1. Lightly coat a large non-stick skillet with cooking spray, heat over medium heat. Add onion & garlic, saute for 4 -5 mins., until onion begins to brown. Add green pepper and carrots. Continue to cook for 8 -10 mins., until soft.
2. Add remaining ingredients (except buns and cheese). Bring to a boil, reduce heat to low and simmer 20 mins., until slightly thickened.
3. Cut buns open, place cut side up on a baking sheet and toast under broiler.
4. Top buns with hot bean mixture and grated cheese. Return to broiler and broil just until cheese melts.

Makes 4 servings.
Exchanges for each serving of 2 bun halves:

3 Starch	1 1/2 Lean meat
1 Vegetable	

49g Carbohydrate, 18g Protein, 8g Fat, 365 cal
(49g available Carbohydrates)

Hot Tamale Pie

1 tsp	Canola oil
1/2 cup	Onions, chopped
1	Green pepper, chopped
1	can (14oz) diced Tomatoes
1	can (14oz) Kidney beans, drained & rinsed
1 1/3 cups	Corn kernels, frozen
1 tbsp	Chili powder
3 cups	Chicken broth (or dehydrated broth & water)
1 1/4 cups	Cornmeal
1/2 cup	Skim milk powder
1 1/2 cups	'Light' Cheddar cheese, grated

1. Preheat oven to 350°F. Lightly coat a 9" baking dish with cooking spray.
2. Heat oil in a large non-stick skillet over medium heat. Add onion and green pepper, cook 4 -5 mins., until tender. Stir in tomatoes, kidney beans, corn, & chili powder. Reduce heat to low and simmer for 15 mins, until thickened.
3. Meanwhile, in a large saucepan stir together broth, cornmeal & skim milk powder. Cook over medium heat stirring frequently until smooth and thickened, 8 -10 mins.
4. Spread cornmeal mixture in the bottom and up the sides of the prepared pan. Pour in the bean mixture. Bake for 40 minutes.
5. Sprinkle with cheese and continue baking for 5 mintues. Cut into 6 squares.

Makes 6 servings.
Exchanges for each serving of 1 square:

1 Starch	3 Vegetable
1/2 Low-fat milk	1 Medium-fat meat
1 Other Carbohydrate	

43g Carbohydrate, 20g Protein, 9g Fat, 354 cal
(43g available Carbohydrates)

Spicy Bean Hot Pot

2 tsp	Olive oil
1/2 cup	Onions, chopped
2 stalks	Celery, chopped
2 cloves	Garlic, minced
1	can (14oz) Stewed tomatoes, with chilies
1	can (5oz) Tomato paste
1 - 2 tsp	Tabasco sauce
1 tsp	Salt
1/2 tsp	Pepper
1	can (14oz) Kidney beans, drained & rinsed
1	can (14oz) Pinto beans, drained & rinsed
1	can (14oz) Cannellini beans, drained & rinsed
1/4 cup	Parsley, chopped

1. Heat the olive oil in a saucepan over medium heat. Add the onion, celery & garlic. Cook, stirring occasionally for 4 - 5 minutes, until vegetables are tender.
2. Stir in the stewed tomatoes, tomato paste, tabasco sauce, salt & pepper. Bring to a boil, reduce heat and simmer for 10 minutes.
3. Add the drained & rinsed beans, cover and simmer for 20 - 25 minutes. Sprinkle with parsley and serve.

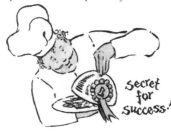

Secret for Success!

Boiling canned beans causes them to split and become mushy. Always add the beans at the end of the cooking time and just let them simmer.

Makes 4 servings.
Exchanges for each serving of 1/4th recipe:
2 1/2 Starch
1 Vegetable
1 1/2 Lean meat

44g Carbohydrates, 18g Protein, 4g Fat, 322 cal
(44g available Carbohydrates)

Idaho Chili stew

1 tsp	Vegetable oil
1/4 cup	Onions, chopped
1 large	Baking potato, peeled & diced
2	Carrots, diced
1 cup	Zucchini, chopped
1	can (19oz) Chickpeas, drained & rinsed
3/4 cup	Lentils, sorted & rinsed
1 cup	Corn, frozen kernels
1	can (14oz) diced Tomatoes
1 cup	Beef (or vegetable) broth, or dehydrated & water
1 cup	Tomato juice
2 tsp	Chili powder
	Optional topping: 'fat-free' sour cream

1. Heat vegetable oil in a large sauce pan over medium heat. Add chopped onion and cook just until softened, 3-4 minutes.
2. Add all remaining ingredients. Bring to a boil, reduce heat. Cover and simmer for 45 - 60 minutes, until lentils are tender.
3. Ladel into bowls and serve. Top with 'fat-free' sour cream if desired.

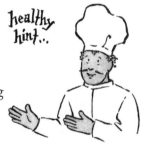

healthy hint...

Lentils are harvested and packaged right from the fields and sometimes contain shrivelled hard beans & debris. Always sort and rinse lentils before cooking

Makes 6 servings.
Exchanges for each serving of 1/6th recipe:
3 Starch   1/2 Very lean meat
1 Vegetable

50g Carbohydrate, 14g protein, 2g Fat, 271 cal
(50g available Carbohydrates)

Texas Red Beans with Rice

2/3 cup	Wild rice, raw
3/4 cup	White long-grain rice, raw
2	Vegetable broth cubes
2 tsp	Olive oil
1/2 cup	Onions, chopped
1	Green or red pepper, chopped
1 clove	Garlic, minced
1	can (14oz) Kidney Beans, rinsed & drained
2 cups	Peas & carrots, frozen
1 tsp	Salt
1/2 tsp	Oregano, dried
1/2 tsp	Thyme, dried
1/2 tsp	Tabasco sauce

1. Add wild rice and broth cubes to 3 cups of water in a large saucepan. Bring to a boil over high heat. Reduce heat to low, cover and simmer for 25 minutes.
2. Stir white rice into wild rice. Cover and continue to simmer for 20 minutes.
3. Meanwhile, in a large non-stick skillet, heat olive oil over medium heat. Saute onions, pepper, & garlic until softened, 5 - 6 mins. Reduce heat to low and add remaining ingredients. Simmer 15 minutes, stirring occasionally.
4. Serve bean mixture over rice.

time for
a change

For authentic 'Red beans & Rice' substitute frozen Okra for the peas. Also, wild rice should rinsed & sorted like lentils (see page 115).

Makes 6 servings.
Exchanges for each serving of 1/6th recipe:
3 Starch
2 Vegetable

55g Carbohydrate, 12g Protein, 3g Fat, 321 cal
(55g available Carbohydrates)

Risotto Primavera

1 tbsp	Butter
2 stalks	Celery, thinly sliced
1 cup	Mushrooms, thinly sliced
1/4 cup	Green onions, chopped
2 cloves	Garlic, minced
1 cup	White rice (Arborio), raw
1	can (10oz) Chicken broth, concentrated
1/2 cup	Peas, frozen
1/2 cup	Zucchini, shredded
1/4 cup	Parmesan cheese, shredded

1. Melt butter in a large saucepan (or a deep skillet). Add celery, mushrooms, green onions & garlic. Saute 5-6 minutes, until tender. Add the uncooked rice, cook and stir for 2 minutes, until lightly toasted.
2. Add the chicken broth, 1 1/2cup of water and a dash of salt & pepper. Bring to a boil, reduce heat, cover and simmer for 25 minutes without peeking.
3. Stir in peas, zucchini, & parmesan cheese. Remove from heat and let stand covered for 5 minutes. Serve immediately.

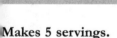
Make it Special

Although you can use ordinary white rice and grated parmesan; Arborio (Italian rice) and freshly shredded parmesan make it special.

Makes 5 servings.
Exchanges for each serving of 1/5th recipe:

2 Starch	1/2 Fat
1 Vegetable	

35g Carbohydrate, 9g Protein, 5g Fat, 231 cal
(35g available Carbohydrates)

Tortilla Mancotti

12	6" Corn tortillas
1	pkg (10oz) frozen Spinach, thawed & drained
2 cups	Cottage cheese, 1%
1/3 cup	Parmesan cheese, grated
1	Egg
1/2 tsp	Salt
1/4 tsp	Pepper
1/4 tsp	Nutmeg, ground
1	can (14oz)Tomato sauce, with onions, peppers & celery
1 tsp	Italian seasoning
1/2 tsp	Garlic powder
1 cup	Part skim Mozzarella cheese, grated

1. Preheat oven to 375°F. Wrap tortillas in foil; heat in oven for 10 minutes.
2. Drain spinach well in a colander and squeeze out excess moisture. Combine with cottage cheese, parmesan, egg, salt, pepper, & nutmeg in a mixing bowl.
3. In a separate bowl stir together the tomato sauce, Italian seasoning, & garlic powder. Spread half of the tomato sauce in a 9 x 13" baking dish.
4. Spoon about 1/4 cup of the spinach mixture down the center of each tortilla. Roll up and place seam side down on the tomato sauce. Spread with remaining tomato sauce and sprinkle with mozzarella.
5. Cover with foil and bake for 30 minutes, uncover and bake for 5 minutes.

Makes 4 servings.
Exchanges for each serving of 3 tortillas:
2 Starch   4 Lean meat
1 Vegetable

32g Carbohydrate, 35g Protein, 11g Fat, 433 cal
(32g available Carbohydrates)

Pasta Shells Florentine

24	Jumbo pasta shells
1	pkg (10oz) frozen Spinach, thawed & squeezed dry
2 cups	Part skim Mozzarella cheese, grated
1 1/2 cups	Cottage cheese (1%)
3	Green onions, chopped
2	Egg whites
1/4 cup	Parmesan cheese, grated
1/4 tsp	Nutmeg, ground
1	can (14oz) Marinara sauce (or 1 3/4 cups bottled)

1. Cook shells according to package instructions. Drain, handling carefully so as not to break them. Set aside. Preheat oven to 350°F.
2. In a large mixing bowl combine well-drained spinach, 1 cup mozzarella, cottage cheese, green onions, egg whites, parmesan & nutmeg.
3. Fill each shell with the cheese mixture and place in a 9 x 13" baking dish. Spoon Marinara sauce around shells. Cover with foil.
4. Bake 35 minutes. Sprinkle with remaining mozzarella and return to oven. Continue to bake, uncovered, for 5 minutes.

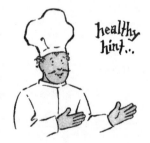

healthy hint...

Be a label sleuth! You can use any tomato sauce for this recipe but Marinara sauce has less fat than most other canned tomato sauces.

Makes 6 servings.
Exchanges each serving of 4 shells:

1 1/2 Starch	1 Vegetable
1/2 Low-fat milk	2 1/2 Lean meat

33g Carbohydrate, 28g Protein, 11g Fat, 352 cal
(33 g available Carbohydrates)

Scalloped Noodles

8 ounce	Egg noodles, medium
1 tsp	Butter
1/3 cup	Onions, chopped
1	Red pepper, chopped
2 cups	Mushrooms, sliced
1	can (10oz) Cream of mushroom soup, '1/2 fat'
1/2 cup	Milk, 1%
3/4 cup	'Light' sour cream
1/2 tsp	Pepper
2 tsp	Worcestershire sauce
1 cup	Corn Flake® crumbs
3/4 cup	'Light' Cheddar cheese, grated

1. Preheat oven to 350°F. Lightly coat a 9 x 13" casserole with cooking spray. Cook noodles as directed on package, drain and set aside.
2. Melt 1 tsp butter in a large non-stick skillet. Add onion, red pepper & mushrooms, cook over medium heat until tender, about 5 mins. Remove from heat. Stir in mushroom soup, milk, sour cream, worcestershire sauce & pepper.
3. Gently stir soup mixture into noodles. Spoon into prepared casserole dish.
4. Combine cornflake crumbs and cheese. Sprinkle over noodle mixture.
5. Bake for 30 minutes, until heated through.

Makes 6 servings.
Exchanges for each serving of 1/6th recipe:

2 Starch	1/2 Lean meat
1 Vegetable	1 Fat

34g Carbohydrate, 12g Protein, 8g Fat, 267 cal
(34g available Carbohydrates)

Mushroom & Spinach Lasagna

12	Spinach lasagna noodles
1	Onion, chopped
1	Green pepper, chopped
2 cloves	Garlic, minced
2	cans (14oz) tomato sauce
2 tsp	Italian seasoning
1 cup	Zucchini, diced
1 1/2 cups	Mushrooms, sliced
1	pkg (10oz) Spinach, thawed & squeezed dry
1 1/2 cups	Ricotta cheese
2	Egg whites
1 cup	Part skim Mozzarella cheese, grated
1/4 cup	Parmesan cheese, grated

1. Coat a large non-stick skillet with cooking spray and preheat over medium heat. Add onion, peppers & garlic. Cook 4 - 5 minutes, until softened. Add tomatoes, seasoning, zucchini & mushrooms. Bring to a boil, reduce heat and simmer, uncovered 20 minutes. Preheat oven to 350°F.
2. Meanwhile, cook noodles as directed on the package, rinse and drain well.
3. Combine ricotta, egg whites, and well-drained spinach in a mixing bowl.
4. Spread 1/2 cup tomato sauce in a 9 x 13" baking dish. Top with 4 noodles, overlapping to fit. Layer with half of the ricotta mixture, a third of the tomato sauce, and half of the mozzarella. Repeat layers. Top with the last four noodles, and the remaining tomato sauce. Cover loosely with foil.
5. Bake for 40 mins. Uncover, sprinkle with parmesan and bake 10 mins.

Makes 8 servings.
Exchanges for each serving of 1/8th recipe:
2 1/2 Starch   2 Medium-fat meat
1 Vegetable

44g Carbohydrate, 22g Protein, 10g Fat, 365 cal
(44g available Carbohydrates)

Potato Pizza

2 lbs	Red potatoes
1/2 tsp	Salt
2	Egg whites
1/2 tsp	Pepper
1/4 tsp	Part skim Mozzarella cheese, grated
2 cloves	Garlic, minced
2 cups	Zucchini, grated
1 1/2 cups	Onion, diced
1/2 cup	Tomatoes, chopped
12	Black olives, sliced
2	Fresh Basil, snipped
1 tbsp	Fresh Oregano, snipped
1/2 cup	Feta cheese, crumbled

1. Thinly slice potatoes into a large bowl of salted cold water, set aside. For a crispy crust, the potatoes should be as thin as possible.
2. Preheat oven to 375°F and coat a pizza pan with cooking spray.
3. Drain potatoes and pat dry. Gently toss with egg white, & pepper. Arrange potatoes in concentric circles around the pizza pan, overlapping, until the pan is covered and the potatoes are all used up.
4. Sprinkle with the grated mozzarella cheese, the minced garlic, zucchini, onion, tomatoes, & olives.
5. Bake for 45 - 50 minutes until potatoes are tender and crispy. Sprinkle with basil, oregano & feta; cook for another 5 minutes. Cut into 8 wedges to serve.

Makes 8 servings.
Each serving of 1 wedge:
2 Starch   2 Lean meat
1 Vegetable

35g Carbohydrate, 18g Protein, 11g Fat, 304 cal
(35 g available Carbohydrates)

Cookies & Bars

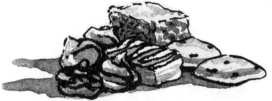

	Page

Oatmeal Raisin Cookies

1/2 cup	Margarine, melted
1/3 cup	Brown sugar
2	Eggs
1 tsp	Vanilla extract
1 cup	Raisins
1 1/2 cups	Rolled oats
3/4 cup	All purpose flour
1/3 cup	Splenda®
1 tsp	Baking powder
1 tsp	Cinnamon
1/4 tsp	Baking soda
1/4 tsp	Salt

1. Preheat oven to 375°F.
2. With an electric mixer beat the melted margarine, brown sugar, eggs, and vanilla together until smooth.
3. In a separate bowl combine the remaining ingredients.
4. Stir the dry ingredients into the margarine mixture until well blended.
5. Drop by heaping spoonfuls 1 1/2" apart on a cookie sheet.
6. Bake for 8 - 10 minutes, until lightly browned. Makes 48 cookies.

chef's secret...

Low fat cookies taste best served warm from the oven or reheated briefly in the microwave.

Makes 24 servings.
Exchanges for each serving of 2 cookies:
1 Starch
1 Fat

14g Carbohydrate, 2g Protein, 5g fat, 105 cal
(14g available Carbohydrates)

Peanut Butter Cookies

1/2 cup	Margarine, softened
3/4 cup	Brown sugar
1 tsp	Vanilla extract
1 cup	'Fat-reduced' peanut butter
2	Eggs
1 1/4 cup	All purpose flour
1 cup	Bran, 100%
3/4 cup	Rolled oats
1/2 cup	Splenda®
2 tsp	Baking soda

1. Preheat oven to 350°F.
2. With an electric mixer beat the margarine, brown sugar, vanilla, peanut butter & eggs together until light and creamy.
3. In a separate bowl combine the flour, bran, rolled oats, Splenda® & baking soda.
4. Stir the dry ingredients into the margarine mixture until well blended.
5. Drop by heaping spoonfuls 1 1/2" apart on a cookie sheet.
6. Bake for 15 -18 minutes. Makes 60 cookies.

If you are modifying cookie recipes, substitute Splenda® for the white sugar only. Using some brown sugar results in a nicer chewy texture. *Secret for Success!*

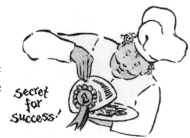

Makes 30 servings.
Exchanges for each serving of 2 cookies:
1 Starch
1 Fat

14g Carbohydrate, 3g Protein, 7g Fat, 126 cal
(14g available Carbohydrates)

Chocolate Ginger Cookies

1/2 cup	Margarine, softened
1/3 cup	Fancy molasses
1/2 cup	Cocoa powder
1 tsp	Vanilla extract
1 1/2 cups	All purpose flour
1/3 cup	Splenda®
1 tsp	Baking soda
1 tsp	Cinnamon
1/2 tsp	Ginger, ground
1 tsp	Salt
2 tbsp	White sugar

1. Preheat oven to 350°F.
2. With an electric mixer beat together the margarine, molasses, cocoa & vanilla until well blended.
3. In a separate bowl combine the flour with the Splenda®, baking soda, cinnamon, ginger & salt.
4. Beat the dry ingredients into the margarine mixture just until blended.
5. Form dough into 36 balls. Dip tops into granulated sugar and place 1" apart on an ungreased baking sheet.
6. Bake for 8 - 9 minutes, until tops are puffed and cracked.

Makes 18 servings.
Exchanges for each serving of 2 cookies:
1 Starch
1 Fat

15g Carbohydrate, 2g Protein, 6g Fat, 116 cal
(15g available Carbohydrates)

Oatmeal Chocolate Chip Cookies

1/4 cup	Margarine, softened
1/4 cup	Brown sugar
1	Egg
2 tbsp	Corn syrup
1/2 tsp	Vanilla extract
1 cup	All purpose flour
1/4 cup	Skim milk powder
1/4 cup	Splenda®
1/2 tsp	Baking soda
1/4 tsp	Salt
3/4 cup	Rolled oats
1/2 cup	Crispy rice cereal
1/2 cup	Semi sweet chocolate chips

1. Preheat oven to 350°F.
2. Beat the margarine and brown sugar together with an electric mixer on high speed, until light and fluffy. Add egg, corn syrup & vanilla, beat well.
3. In a separate bowl stir together the flour, skim milk powder, Splenda®, baking soda & salt.
4. With electric mixer on low speed, blend dry ingredients into the margarine mixture. Stir in rolled oats, chocolate chips, & crispy rice cereal.
5. Drop by spoonfuls, 2" apart, on an ungreased cookie sheet.
6. Bake for 10 minutes or until lightly browned. Makes 44 cookies.

Makes 22 servings.
Exchanges for each serving of 2 cookies:
1 Starch
1/2 Fat

14g Carbohydrate, 2g Protein, 4g Fat, 98 cal
(14g available Carbohydrates)

Walnut Crescents

3/4 cup	Unsalted butter, softened
1/3 cup	Confectioners' sugar
1/2 cup	Splenda®
1 1/4 cups	All purpose flour
1/2 cup	Cornstarch
1/3 cup	Walnuts, finely chopped
1/2 tsp	Vanilla extract
2 tbsp	Confectioners' sugar

1. Preheat oven to 325°F.
2. Finely chop walnuts in a food processor. Spread on a baking sheet and toast in preheated oven for 5 minutes. Let cool.
3. In a large mixing bowl beat butter and 1/3 cup confectioners' sugar with an electric mixer on medium until blended. Increase speed to high and continue beating until light and fluffy.
4. Stir in remaining ingredients. Knead with hands until mixture forms a ball. Roll scant tablespoons of dough into 50 crescent shapes. Place on ungreased cookie sheet 1" apart.
5. Bake 15 minutes, until edges begin to brown. Remove to wire rack to cool.
6. When completely cool, dust with 2 Tbsp sifted confectioners' sugar.

Makes 25 servings.
Exchanges for each serving of 2 cookies:
1/2 Starch
1 Fat

10g Carbohydrate, 1g Protein, 6g Fat, 98 cal
(10g available Carbohydrates)

Lemon Cookies

1/2 cup	Margarine, softened
1/3 cup	Granulated sugar
1	Egg
1 tbsp	Lemon peel
2 tbsp	Lemon juice
1 tsp	Vanilla extract
1 1/4 cup	All purpose flour
1/2 tsp	Baking powder
1/4 tsp	Baking soda
1/3 cup	Splenda®
1 tbsp	White sugar

1. Preheat oven to 350°F.
2. Beat margarine and sugar together on high speed until light and fluffy. Beat in egg, lemon peel, lemon juice & vanilla extract.
3. In a separate bowl stir together the flour, baking powder, baking soda, & Splenda®. Add dry ingredients to the margarine mixture, beat until blended.
4. Drop by rounded teaspoonfuls onto cookie sheet 1 1/2" apart. Press flat with a fork that has been dipped in sugar making a criss-cross pattern.
5. Bake 10-11 minutes, until edges are lightly browned. Makes 36 cookies.

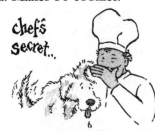

chef's secret...

To squeeze the most from a lemon or lime, grate off the peel, then roll the fruit on the counter with your hand and **then** juice it.

Makes 18 servings.
Exchanges for each serving of 2 cookies:
1 Starch
1 Fat

11g Carbohydrate, 1g Protein, 6g Fat, 102 cal
(11g available Carbohydrates)

Fruit & Nut Drops

2 1/4 cups	All purpose flour
2 tsp	Baking powder
1/2 cup	Splenda®
1/2 tsp	Salt
3/4 cup	Margarine, softened
1/2 cup	Brown sugar
2	Eggs
2 tbsp	Milk, 1%
1 tsp	Vanilla extract
1 cup	Dates, finely chopped
1/2 cup	Walnuts, chopped
1/4 cup	Maraschino cherries, chopped
2 cups	Corn Flakes® crushed
18	Maraschino cherries, quartered

1. Preheat oven to 350°F.
2. With an electric mixer beat the margarine and brown sugar together until light and fluffy. Add the eggs, one at a time, beating well after each addition.
3. In a separate bowl combine the flour, baking powder, Splenda®, & salt.
4. With the mixer on low, gradually add the dry ingredients to the margarine mixture, until well blended. Stir in dates, walnuts, & chopped cherries.
5. Shape spoonfuls of the dough into 72 balls and roll in the crushed Corn Flakes®. Place 1 1/2" apart on cookie sheets. Make an indent in each cookie and top with a cherry quarter.
6. Bake for 10 -12 minutes, until lightly browned.

Makes 36 servings.
Exchanges for each serving of 2 cookies:
1 Starch
1 Fat

15g Carbohydrate, 2g Protein, 5g Fat, 112 cal
(15g available Carbohydrates)

Cherry Almond Macaroons

2 1/2 cups	Unsweetened coconut
1/2 cup	Candied Cherries, chopped
1/4 cup	Almonds, ground
1/3 cup	White sugar
1/4 cup	All purpose flour
1/4 tsp	Salt
4	Egg whites

1. Preheat oven to 325°F. Line a large baking sheet with cooking parchment or foil.
2. In a medium mixing bowl stir together coconut, cherries, almonds, sugar, flour, and salt. Stir in egg whites until well mixed.
3. Drop mixture in 48 mounds, onto prepared cookie sheet. Moisten hands and shape mounds into balls.
4. Bake cookies for 25 minutes or until lightly browned.

Black & White Macaroons:

Follow the above recipe but delete the cherries & almonds and increase the coconut by 1/4 cup. Shape the mounds into ovals and flatten slightly. Bake as above. Melt 2 squares of semi sweet baking chocolate and 2 tsp. butter in a double boiler (or microwave). Dip half of each baked and cooled cookie into the melted chocolate so that half is chocolate and half is white. Let dry on waxed paper. Makes 48 cookies.

Cherry Almond Macaroons
Makes 48 servings.
Each serving of 1 cookie:
1/2 Starch
1/2 Fat

Black & White Macaroons
Each serving of 1 cookie:
1/2 Vegetable
1 Fat
(3g carbohydrate, 1g protein, 4g fat, 51cal)

4g Carbohydrate, 1g Protein, 4g Fat, 52 cal
(4g available Carbohydrates)

Butterscotch Crisps

1/4 cup	Margarine
4 cups	Miniature marshmallows
1/2 cup	Butterscotch chips
5 cups	Special K cereal®
1/2 cup	Peanuts, dry-roasted, chopped
1/2 cup	Raisins
1/4 cup	Wheat germ

1. Spread waxed paper onto 2 baking sheets and set aside.
2. In a large heavy saucepan, melt margarine over medium-low heat. Add marshmallows; cook and stir until melted. Stir in butterscotch chips. Cook and stir until melted and smooth. Remove from heat.
3. Stir in Special K cereal®, peanuts, raisins, and wheat germ. Drop by spoonfuls onto waxed paper into 72 mounds. Let cool.

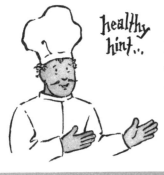

healthy hint... Fiber has many health benefits and it is especially an important part of a diabetic diet because it slows the digestion of food thus allowing blood glucose levels to rise more slowly. Sneak more fiber into your diet with snacks such as this recipe.

Makes 36 servings.
Exchanges for each serving of 2 crisps:
1 Starch

12g Carbohydrate, 1g protein, 2g fat, 73 cal
(12g available Carbohydrates)

Peanut Butter & Banana Bars

1	Egg
2	Bananas, mashed
1/2 cup	'Reduced-fat' peanut butter
1 cup	Rolled oats
1/2 cup	Coconut, unsweetened
1/3 cup	Sesame seeds
1/4 cup	Raisins
2 tbsp	Brown sugar

1. Preheat oven to 350°F. Lightly coat an 8" square baking pan with cooking spray.
2. In a large mixing bowl beat the egg, bananas & peanut butter with an electric mixer until creamy.
3. Add the remaining ingredients and stir until well blended. Spread in the prepared pan and bake for 25 minutes, until edges pull away from the sides of the pan.
4. Cool on a wire rack. Cut into 16 squares to serve.

Vary these bars with your own favorite combination of dried fruit & nuts. Try currants, dates, dried cranberries or snipped apricots, sunflower or pumpkin seeds or...

time for a change

Makes 16 servings.
Exchanges for each serving of 1 square:
1 Starch
1 Fat

13g Carbohydrate, 4g Protein, 7g Fat, 126 cal
(13g available Carbohydrates)

Brownie Brittle

1/3 cup	Unsalted butter
1 square	Semi sweet chocolate
1/2 tsp	Ginger, ground
1/2 tsp	Cinnamon
1/4 cup	Brown sugar
1/4 cup	White sugar
1	Egg, beaten with a fork
1 tsp	Vanilla extract
1/2 cup	All purpose flour
1/2 cup	Almonds, ground

1. Preheat oven to 375°F.
2. Melt butter in a large saucepan over medium-low heat. Add chocolate, ginger & cinnamon. When the chocolate starts to melt remove from heat and stir until completely melted.
3. Stir in brown sugar, white sugar, vanilla, & egg. Beat with a wooden spoon until smooth. Add flour & stir to blend completely.
4. Pour batter onto an ungreased 10 x 15" jelly roll pan. Spread the batter with a rubber spatula into a thin, even layer over the bottom of the pan. Sprinkle with ground almonds.
5. Bake for 8 -10 minutes, until set. Cool for 20 minutes. Cut into 36 rough shaped, equal size pieces, resembling nut brittle.

Makes 18 servings.
Exchanges for each serving of 2 pieces:
1/2 Starch
1 Fat

8g Carbohydrate, 2g Protein, 7g Fat, 98 cal
(8g available Carbohydrates)

S'more Brownies

1/2 cup	Cocoa powder
1/3 cup	Brown sugar
1/2 cup	Splenda®
1/4 cup	All purpose flour
1/2 tsp	Baking powder
3	Eggs
1/4 cup	Vegetable oil
2 tsp	Vanilla extract
3/4 cup	Marshmallows, miniature
6	Graham crackers, broken into small pieces

1. Preheat oven to 350°F. Line a 8" square baking pan with foil large enough so that the ends extend on two sides. Coat with cooking spray.
2. In a large mixing bowl stir together the cocoa, brown sugar, Splenda®, flour & baking powder. Beat the eggs, oil & vanilla together in a separate bowl.
3. Add the egg mixture to the dry ingredients and stir until blended.
4. Fold in 1/2 cup each of the miniature marshmallows and the graham cracker bits. Spread evenly in the prepared pan. Bake 10 minutes.
5. Sprinkle with the remaining marshmallows and graham cracker bits. Press gently to partially submerge into the batter. Continue to bake for 20 minutes longer, until top marshmallows are golden. Cool completely in pan.
6. Lift foil by ends onto a cutting board, peel off foil, and cut into 16 squares.

Makes 16 servings.
Exchanges for each serving of 1 square:
1/2 Starch
1 Fat

11g Carbohydrate, 2g Protein, 5g Fat, 86 cal
(11g available Carbohydrates)

Peanut Butter Granola Bars

3/4 cup	Whole-wheat flour
1/4 cup	Splenda®
1/2 tsp	Baking soda
3/4 cup	'Reduced-fat' peanut butter
1/2 cup	Margarine
1/3 cup	Brown sugar
1 tsp	Vanilla extract
2	Eggs
1/2 cup	Applesauce, unsweetened
1 3/4 cups	Rolled oats
1/4 cup	Wheat germ
1/3 cup	Mini chocolate chips
1/4 cup	Dry roasted peanuts, chopped

1. Preheat oven to 350°F. Lightly coat a 13 x 9" baking pan with cooking spray and dust with flour, set aside.
2. Combine the whole wheat flour, Splenda® & baking soda in a small bowl.
3. With a electric mixer beat the peanut butter and margarine on medium speed until softened. Add the brown sugar and vanilla, beat until well blended. Add the eggs, one at a time, beating well after each addition.
4. On low speed, stir in the applesauce. Add the flour mixture and stir until well blended. Stir in the rolled oats, wheat germ, chocolate chips & peanuts. Spread in the prepared baking pan.
5. Bake for 25 minutes or until a toothpick inserted in the centre comes out clean. Cool completely in the pan on a wire rack. Cut into 24 bars.

Makes 24 servings.
Exchanges for each serving of 1 bar:
1 Starch
1 1/2 Fat

14g Carbohydrate, 4g Protein, 8g Fat, 142 cal
(14g available Carbohydrates)

Zucchini Snacking Cake

1 1/4 cups	All purpose flour
1/2 cup	Brown sugar
1/2 cup	Splenda®
2 tbsp	Cocoa powder
1 1/2 tsp	Baking powder
1 tsp	Cinnamon
1/4 tsp	Salt
1/4 cup	Vegetable oil
2	Eggs
2	Egg whites
1 tsp	Vanilla extract
1 cup	Zucchini, shredded
1/3 cup	Raisins
1/2 cup	Mini chocolate chips

1. Preheat oven to 350°F. Lightly coat a 9 x 9" cake pan with cooking spray.
2. Combine flour, brown sugar, Splenda®, cocoa, baking powder, cinnamon, & salt in a large mixing bowl. In a separate bowl beat together the oil, eggs, egg whites, & vanilla. Add the egg mixture, raisins, & zucchini to the dry ingredients. Stir just until blended.
3. Pour into the prepared pan and bake for 30 minutes, until the top springs back when lightly pressed.
4. Sprinkle with chocolate chips and let sit for 5 mins. Spread melted chips gently to cover the cake. Let cool on a wire rack.

Makes 16 servings.
Exchanges for each serving of 1 square:
1/2 Starch   1 Fat
1 Fruit

23g Carbohydrate, 3g protein, 6g Fat, 153kcal
(23g available Carbohydrates)

Marbled Cheesecake Squares

20	Vanilla wafers, small
2 tbsp	Confectioners' sugar
3 tbsp	Cocoa powder
3 tbsp	Margarine, melted
2 squares	Semi-sweet chocolate
16 oz	'Light' cream cheese
1/2 cup	Splenda®
1/2 tsp	Vanilla extract
2	

1. Preheat oven to 350°F. Lightly coat a 9 x 9" baking pan with cooking spray
2. Crush vanilla wafers with a rolling pin. Mix together the wafer crumbs, icing sugar, cocoa, & margarine. Press firmly onto the bottom of prepared pan.
3. Melt chocolate in the microwave or in a double boiler. Let cool slightly.
4. Beat cream cheese, Splenda®, vanilla & eggs until creamy and well blended. Stir half of the cream cheese mixture into the melted chocolate.
5. Spoon dollops of the white and chocolate batters over prepared crust. Gently swirl a knife through the batters being careful not to disturb the crust.
6. Bake 40-45 minutes, until set. Cool. Refrigerate for at least 3 hours (or overnight). Cut into 16 squares to serve.

Make it Special

For a pretty presentation; cut whole strawberries in very thin slices without cutting all the way through. Spread into fan shape. Top each square with a fanned strawberry. Drizzle with 'light' chocolate sundae sauce.

Makes 16 servings.
Exchanges for each serving of 1 square:

1/2 Starch	1 Fat
1/2 High-fat meat	

7g Carbohydrate, 4g Protein, 10g fat, 136 cal
(7g available Carbohydrates)

Desserts

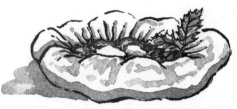

Carrot Cake

2 cups	All purpose flour
2/3 cup	Splenda®
2 tsp	Baking powder
1 tsp	Baking soda
1 tsp	Cinnamon
1 tsp	Salt
6	Egg whites
1/2 cup	Granulated sugar
1/2 cup	Applesauce, unsweetened
1/2 cup	Plain Yogurt, low fat
1/4 cup	Vegetable oil
1 tsp	Vanilla Extract
2 cups	Carrots, grated
1/2 cup	Walnuts, chopped
1 cup	Pineapple, crushed, drained

1. Preheat oven to 350°F. Lightly coat a 9 x 13" baking pan with cooking spray. Combine the first 6 ingredients in a medium-sized mixing bowl.
2. In a separate mixing bowl beat the egg whites until soft peaks form. Slowly beat in the sugar. Stir in the applesauce, yogurt, vegetable oil & vanilla.
3. Add the dry ingredients and stir just until combined. Gently fold in the carrots, walnuts & well-drained pineapple.
4. Spread in prepared pan. Bake 50 - 60 minutes, until a toothpick inserted in the centre comes out clean. Cool on a wire rack. When completely cooled frost with cream cheese frosting (pg.159).

Makes 20 servings.
Exchanges for each serving of 1 piece (with icing):

1/2 Starch	1/2 Lean meat
1 Fruit	1 Fat

23g Carbohydrate, 5g Protein, 7g Fat, 173 cal
(23g available Carbohydrates)

Cocoa Berry Bread Pudding

1/4 cup	Almonds, slivered
8 slices	Whole wheat bread
2 cups	Raspberries, fresh or frozen (thawed)
1	Egg
2	Egg whites
1 1/3 cup	Evaporated skim milk
1/4 cup	Cocoa
1/4 cup	Splenda®
2 tbsp	Chocolate or raspberry liquer

1. Preheat oven to 350°F. Lightly coat a 9 x 13" baking pan with cooking spray. Lightly toast almonds for about 5 minutes in preheated oven.
2. Remove crusts from bread slices and discard. Cut bread into small cubes.
3. Spread half of the bread cubes in the prepared pan. Sprinkle with half of the raspberries.
4. In a medium-sized mixing bowl combine the egg, egg whites, evaporated skim milk, cocoa, Splenda® & liquer. Beat until well blended.
5. Pour half of the egg mixture over the bread and raspberries in pan. Top with the remaining bread cubes and raspberries. Pour the remaining egg mixture evenly over all. Sprinkle with toasted almonds.
6. Bake 30 - 35 minutes, until set.

Makes 8 servings.
Exchanges for each serving of 1/8th recipe:

1/2 Starch	1/2 Low-fat milk
1/2 Fruit	1/2 Lean meat

21g Carbohydrate, 9g Protein, 4g Fat, 164 cal
(21g available Carbohydrates)

Pumpkin Pie

1	Frozen unbaked pie crust
1/3 cup	Splenda®
2 tbsp	All purpose flour
1 tsp	Cinnamon
1/2 tsp	Ginger, ground
1/2 tsp	Nutmeg
1/2 tsp	Salt
3	Egg whites
2 cups	Pumpkin, cooked or canned
1	Egg
1 cup	Evaporated skim milk
1/4 cup	Pure Maple syrup

1. Preheat oven to 425°F. Allow pie crust to thaw slightly.
2. Combine the Splenda®, flour, cinnamon, ginger, nutmeg & salt in a small mixing bowl.
3. In a separate bowl beat the egg whites until soft peaks form. Fold in the pumpkin and the Splenda® mixture.
4. Beat the egg, evaporated milk, and maple syrup together until smooth and then fold into the pumpkin mixture. Pour into pie shell.
5. Bake for 15 mins at 425°F. Reduce heat to 350°F and continue baking 40 minutes, until a knife inserted in the center comes out clean.

Makes 8 servings.
Exchanges for each serving of 1 wedge:
1/2 Starch   1 Fruit
1/2 Whole milk

24g Carbohydrate, 6g Protein, 8g Fat, 191 cal
(24g available Carbohydrates)

Two "Sophisticated" Sundaes

Grilled Banana Sundaes

2 tbsp	Rum
2 tbsp	Splenda®
2	Bananas, peeled
2 cups	Vanilla Ice Milk

1. Preheat barbecue to medium heat; oil grill.Cut bananas in half lengthwise.
2. Mix rum & Splenda® in a small bowl. Brush bananas with rum sauce and place on preheated grill. Grill, turning frequently & basting with sauce 6 - 7 minutes, until golden. Cut grilled bananas in half crosswise.
3. Place 2 banana pieces in each dessert dish, top with ice milk & strawberries.

Makes 4 servings.
Exchanges for each serving of 1 sundae:
1/2 Whole Milk   2 Fruit
33g Carbohydrate, 4g Protein, 4g Fat, 189 cal
(33g available Carbohydrates)

Cherries Jubilee Sundaes

1/4 cup	Splenda®
1 tbsp	Cornstarch
1 1/2 cups	Cherries, frozen or canned, unsweetened
2 tbsp	Slivered Almonds, toasted
1 tsp	Almond Extract
2 cups	Vanilla Ice Milk

1. In a small saucepan whisk Splenda®, cornstarch, & 3/4 cup water.
2. Bring to a boil; boil 1 minute. Stir in cherries and almond extract. Let cool.
3. Scoop ice cream into serving bowls. Top with cherries & toasted almonds.

Makes 6 servings.
Exchanges for each serving of 1 sundae:
1 Fruit   1/2 Whole milk
19g Carbohydrate, 3g Protein, 4g Fat, 124 cal
(19g available Carbohydrates)

Apple & Cheddar Pandowdy

8	Apples, peeled & sliced
2 tsp	Lemon juice
2 tbsp	All purpose flour
1 tsp	Cinnamon
1/2 cup	Apple juice
1/2 cup	Splenda®
3/4 cup	All purpose flour
1/4 cup	White sugar
1 tsp	Baking powder
1/4 tsp	Salt
1/4 cup	Butter, cut in small pieces

1. Preheat oven to 375°F. Lightly coat a 9" square pan with cooking spray.
2. Mix apples and lemon juice in a medium sized saucepan. Sprinkle with 2 tbsp flour and cinnamon, toss gently. Add apple juice and Splenda®. Cook over medium heat for 5 minutes. Spoon into prepared pan.
3. Mix 3/4 cup flour, sugar, baking powder & salt in a medium-sized mixing bowl. With a pastry cutter, cut in butter and cheese until coarse crumbs form. Stir in 1/2 cup of water. Drop dough by tablespoonfuls over hot apple filling.
4. Bake for 40-45 minutes, until golden brown.

chef's
secret...

Splenda® works well for sweetening the fruit filling, but leaving some sugar in the batter results in better color and texture.

Makes 8 servings.
Exchanges for each serving of 1/8th recipe:

1 Starch	1 Fat
2 Fruit	

37g Carbohydrate, 4g Protein, 7g Fat, 225 cal
(37g available Carbohydrates)

Apple Galette

1 1/2 cups	All purpose flour
1/2 tsp	Salt
1/3 cup	Unsalted butter, cut in pieces
10	Apples, peeled & thinly sliced
2 tbsp	Lemon juice
1/4 cup	Splenda®
1 tbsp	All purpose flour
1 tsp	Cinnamon
1 tbsp	Butter
1 tbsp	Milk, 1%
1 tbsp	White sugar
	Walnuts, finely chopped

1. To make the pastry: Combine the flour and salt in a mixing bowl. With a pastry cutter cut in unsalted butter until the size of coarse crumbs.
2. With a fork stir in 3-4 Tbsp of cold water, 1 tbsp at a time, until mixture begins to form a ball. Shape into a flat ball, wrap in plastic wrap, refrigerate 30 minutes or more. Preheat oven to 400°F.
3. Toss apple slices with lemon juice. Stir in flour, Splenda®, and cinnamon.
4. On a lightly floured board roll chilled pastry out into a 14" circle. Roll the dough onto the rolling pin, then unroll onto a large baking sheet.
5. Mound apple filling onto pastry, leaving a 2" border. Dot with 1 Tbsp butter. Fold the border up over the apple filling. Brush exposed edge with milk. Sprinkle with sugar and nuts. Bake for 40 minutes, until crust is golden.

Makes 10 servings.
Exchanges for each serving of 1 wedge:
1 Starch   1 1/2 Fat
1 1/2 Fruit

36g Carbohydrate, 3g Protein, 8g Fat, 233 cal
(36g available Carbohydrates)

Easy Apple Crisp

2 cups	Low fat '5 grain' Granola
2 tbsp	All purpose flour
2 tbsp	Butter, cut in small pieces
1 tsp	Cinnamon
6	Apples, peeled & thinly sliced
1/4 cup	Splenda®
2 tbsp	Lemon juice

1. Preheat oven to 375°F. Lightly coat a 9 x 9" baking dish with cooking spray.
2. Measure granola, flour, butter, & cinnamon into a medium sized mixing bowl. Stir together with a fork until blended.
3. Gently toss apples with lemon juice and Splenda®. Spread in prepared baking dish. Sprinkle with granola mixture.
4. Bake for 40-45 minutes, or until top is crisp and golden.

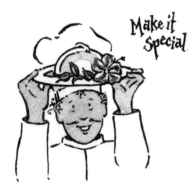

Make it Special

This fast and easy dessert is delicious served warm and topped with a scoop of frozen vanilla yogurt or 'light' ice cream. For Christmas add 1cup of cranberries for a seasonal flavor.

Makes 6 servings.
Exchanges for each serving of 1/6th recipe:
1 Starch   1 Fat
2 Fruit

41g Carbohydrate, 3g protein, 6g fat, 227 cal
(41g available Carbohydrates)

Apple Poundcake

2 1/2 cups	All purpose flour
1/2 cup	Splenda®
1 tbsp	Baking powder
1/4 tsp	Baking soda
1 tsp	Cinnamon
1/2 tsp	Nutmeg
1/2 tsp	Salt
2	Eggs
4	Egg whites
2 tsp	Vanilla extract
1/4 cup	White sugar
1/3 cup	Butter, softened
1/3 cup	Buttermilk, low fat
3	Apples, peeled, cored, & diced
1/3 cup	Walnuts, finely chopped

1. Preheat oven to 350°F. Lightly coat a 10" tube pan with cooking spray. Dust with flour
2. Combine flour, Splenda®, baking powder, baking soda, cinnamon, nutmeg & salt. In a separate bowl whisk together the eggs, egg whites & vanilla.
3. With an electric mixer beat the sugar, butter & buttermilk until creamy.
4. With the electric mixer still running add the dry ingredients alternately with the eggs. Beat until fluffy. Fold in the apples & walnuts.
5. Spread in prepared pan. Bake for 1 hour, until toothpick inserted in center comes out clean. Cool on a wire rack for 10 mins. Remove from pan & cool.

Makes 14 servings.
Exchanges for each serving of 1 slice:
2 Starch   1 Fat
1/2 Fruit

27g Carbohydrate, 5g Protein, 7g Fat, 193 cal
(27g available Carbohydrates)

Apple Turnovers

4	Apples, peeled & chopped
2 tsp	Lemon juice
1/4 cup	Splenda®
1 tbsp	All purpose flour
1/3 cup	Raisins
1/2 tsp	Cinnamon
1/4 tsp	Nutmeg
1/4 tsp	Salt
6 sheets	Phyllo pastry

1. Preheat oven to 400°F. Coat a baking sheet with cooking spray.
2. Combine the chopped apples and lemon juice in a mixing bowl, toss gently. Add Splenda®, flour, raisins, & spices. Toss and set aside.
3. Spread out 1 phyllo sheet at a time. To keep unused phyllo from drying out when working with a sheet, cover with waxed paper and a damp tea towel. Cut phyllo sheet lengthwise into 4 strips, lightly spray with cooking spray.
4. Stack 2 strips on top of each other. Place a heaping spoonful of apple mixture onto bottom of strip, leaving a 1" border. Fold the bottom corner over making a triangle. Continue folding back and forth to form a triangular package. Repeat to make 12 apple filled triangles.
5. Spray turnover tops lightly with cooking spray. Bake for 18 -20 mins. or until golden. Best served warm & crispy from the oven.

Makes 12 servings.
Exchanges for each serving of 1 turnover:
1 Fruit
1 Vegetable

19g Carbohydrate, 1g Protein, .5g fat, 80 cal
(19g available Carbohydrates)

Blueberry Crumble

22	Small Vanilla wafers, crushed
1 tbsp	All purpose flour
2 tbsp	Margarine, melted
1 tbsp	Brown sugar
1/4 tsp	Cinnamon
4 cups	Blueberries, raw or frozen
1/3 cup	Splenda®
2 tbsp	All purpose flour
1 tbsp	Cornstarch
1 tsp	Cinnamon
1/4 tsp	Nutmeg, ground
1/4 tsp	Salt
2 tsp	Lemon juice

1. Preheat oven to 350°F. Lightly coat a 8" baking dish with cooking spray.
2. Crush vanilla wafers in a food processor or with a rolling pin. Combine wafer crumbs with flour, melted margarine, brown sugar, & 1/4 tsp. cinnamon. Set aside.
3. In a large mixing bowl gently toss blueberries with Splenda®, flour, cornstarch & spices. Spoon into prepared baking dish and sprinkle with lemon juice. Spread crumb topping evenly over fruit.
4. Bake for 35 - 40 mins, until top is lightly browned. Best served warm.

Makes 8 servings.
Exchanges for each serving of 1/8th recipe:
1/2 Starch   1/2 Fat
1 Fruit

20g Carbohydrate, 1g Protein, 4g Fat, 119 cal
(20g available Carbohydrates)

Cheesecake Strudel Pie

16 oz	'Light' cream cheese
1/3 cup	Splenda®
1 tsp	Vanilla extract
1	Egg
1 tsp	Lemon peel
6 sheets	Phyllo pastry
1 cup	'Light' sour cream
3 tbsp	Brown sugar
1 tbsp	Lemon juice
24	Strawberries, sliced or whole

1. Preheat oven to 350°F. Lightly coat a deep 9" pie plate with cooking spray.
2. To make the phyllo crust: Cut each phyllo sheet in half to make 12 squares. Using two sheets at a time; lay first 2 sheets in the coated pan & spray with cooking spray. Lay the next two sheets opposite from the first. Spray with cooking spray. Repeat with remaining layers, resulting in edges that hang over the same length all around the pie plate. Spray edges well and then crinkle onto pie plate edge to form an attractive rim.
3. Beat cream cheese, Splenda®, and vanilla until smooth. Beat in egg and lemon peel. Pour into the phyllo crust. Bake for 30 minutes.
4. Mix the sour cream, brown sugar, and lemon juice and pour on cheesecake. Return to oven and bake for 5 minutes. Allow to cool on rack.
5. When pie is completely cool, top with fresh strawberries.

Makes 8 servings.
Each serving of 1 wedge:

1 Starch	1 Lean meat
1/2 Fruit	2 Fat

24g Carbohydrate, 10g Protein, 13g Fat, 266 cal
(24g available Carbohydrates)

Double Chocolate Cupcakes

1 1/2 cups	All purpose flour
1/4 cup	Cocoa powder
1/2 cup	Splenda®
1 tsp	Baking soda
1/2 tsp	Salt
1/2 cup	Orange juice
3 tbsp	Vegetable oil
1	Egg
1 tbsp	Vinegar
1 tsp	Vanilla extract
1/3 cup	Mini chocolate chips
1 tbsp	Confectioner's sugar

1. Preheat oven to 375°F. Line 12 muffin cups with paper liners.
2. In a medium-sized mixing bowl combine the first 5 ingredients.
3. In a separate bowl combine 1/3 cup of water, orange juice, oil, egg, vinegar & vanilla. Make a well in the center of the dry ingredients and pour in the orange juice mixture. Stir just until moistened. Fold in chocolate chips.
4. Spoon into prepared muffin cups. Bake for 12 minutes, or until a toothpick inserted in the center comes out clean. Remove from pan.
5. When cool sprinkle with confectioner's sugar.

Do not overmix the batter or the cupcakes will become chewy and full of tunnels.

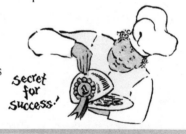

Secret for Success!

Makes 12 servings.
Exchanges for each serving of 1 cupcake:
1 Starch   1 Fat
1/2 Other Carbohydrate

20g Carbohydrate, 3g Protein, 6g Fat, 143 cal
(20g available Carbohydrates)

Lazy Day Peach Pie

1/3 cup	Splenda®
4 tsp	All purpose flour
1/2 tsp	Cinnamon
1/4 tsp	Nutmeg
10	Fresh peaches, peeled & sliced
1 tbsp	Lemon juice
1 envelope	Betty Crocker® piecrust mix
4 tsp	Granulated sugar
2	Egg whites

1. Preheat oven to 375°F. Line a cookie sheet with foil and sprinkle lightly with flour. Make one large pie crust using 1 envelope (enough for a 2 crust pie) and following the directions on the package.
2. Roll pastry out into a 15" circle. Roll onto rolling pin and then unroll onto prepared baking sheet.
3. In a large mixing bowl toss peach slices with Splenda®, flour & spices.
4. Spoon peach mixture onto the crust leaving a 2" border. Sprinkle with lemon juice. Gently fold the border up and over the peaches. Beat the egg whites, then brush on the outside edge of the pie crust. Sprinkle with sugar.
5. Bake for 40-50 minutes, until crust is golden. Let cool on baking sheet. Serve warm or at room temperature.

Makes 10 servings.
Exchanges for each serving of 1 wedge:

1 Starch	1 1/2 Fat
1 Fruit	

25g Carbohydrate, 3g Protein, 9g Fat, 193 cal
(25g available Carbohydrates)

Peach Almond Kuchen

1/2 cup	All purpose flour
2 tbsp	Brown sugar
1/2 tsp	Cinnamon
2 tbsp	Butter
1/4 cup	Almonds, slivered
10	Peaches, peeled & sliced
3 oz	'Light' cream cheese
2	Eggs
1/4 cup	Splenda®
1/4 cup	All purpose flour
1 cup	Buttermilk, low fat

1. Preheat oven to 375°F. Lightly coat a 9 x 9" baking dish with cooking spray. Spread peeled & sliced peaches in prepared pan.
2. Make crumb topping: Stir together the 1/2 cup flour, brown sugar, & cinnamon. With a pastry cutter cut in butter until mixture resembles fine crumbs. Stir in almonds. Set aside.
3. In a medium sized mixing bowl beat cream cheese with an electric mixer. Add buttermilk, eggs, Splenda® & 1/4 cup flour, beat until smooth. Pour over fruit. Sprinkle crumb topping evenly over all.
4. Bake for 30-35 mins, until the filling is set. Cut into 8 squares. Serve warm.

Makes 8 servings.
Exchanges for each serving of 1 square:

1 Starch	1/2 Lean meat
1 Fruit	1 Fat

25g Carbohydrate, 7g Protein, 9g Fat, 209kcal
(25g available Carbohydrates)

Poached Pears with Sherbet

3	Pears
1 tsp	Lemon juice
1/2 cup	White wine
1/4 cup	Apple juice
1 1/2 cups	Raspberry sherbet
1 square	Semisweet chocolate

1. Peel and core pears, cut in half lengthwise; brush with lemon juice.
2. Combine wine and apple juice in a large saucepan, bring to a boil. Reduce heat to low.
3. Carefully add pears, cover and simmer for 15 mins, turning once. Remove from heat, cover and cool for 1 hour.
4. Melt chocolate in the top of a double boiler or microwave. Transfer pears with a slotted spoon, cut-side up, to dessert plates. Top each pear with 1/4 cup sherbet. Drizzle attractively with chocolate.

What's the difference between sorbet & sherbet? Sorbet is a intensely flavored frozen mixture of a sweetened liquid such as fruit juice. Sherbet is like sorbet but it contains milk fat & sometimes gelatin.

Makes 6 servings.
Exchanges for each serving of 1 pear half:
2 Fruit
1 Fat

29g Carbohydrate, 1g Protein, 3g Fat, 164 cal
(29g available Carbohydrates)

Rhubarb Cobbler

3 tbsp	Cornstarch
1 cup	Apple juice
2/3 cup	Splenda®
2 lb	Rhubarb, raw or frozen, diced
1 cup	All purpose flour
1/4 cup	White sugar (divided)
1 1/2 tsp	Baking powder
2 tbsp	Margarine
1/3 cup	Milk, 1%
1 tsp	Cinnamon

1. Preheat oven to 425°F.
2. In a large saucepan combine cornstarch and 1/4 cup of water. Whisk in another 3/4 cup of water & apple juice. Place over medium heat and bring to a boil stirring occasionally. Stir in Splenda® and rhubarb. Return to a boil, reduce heat and simmer for 5 minutes or until rhubarb is tender and mixture is thickened. Pour into a 9"square baking dish.
3. Combine flour, 2 Tbsp sugar & baking powder in a mixing bowl. Cut in margarine with a pastry cutter. Add milk, stir just until moistened. Spoon in mounds on hot rhubarb mixture. Sprinkle with 2 Tbsp sugar & cinnamon.
4. Bake for 20-25 minutes, until topping is lightly browned & cooked through.

Makes 9 servings.
Exchanges for each serving of 1/9th recipe:
1 Starch   1/2 Fat
1 Fruit

29g Carbohydrate, 3g Protein, 3g Fat, 144 cal
(29g available Carbohydrates)

Strawberry Lemon Cream Parfaits

1/3 cup	Splenda®
2 tbsp	Cornstarch
3/4 cup	Milk, 1%
2	Eggs
2 tbsp	Lemon juice
2 tsp	Lemon peel, raw
1/2 cup	'Light' sour cream
1 1/2 cups	Strawberries, sliced

1. Mix Splenda® and cornstarch in a small saucepan. Whisk in milk until smooth. Continue to stir while heating over medium-high heat until boiling. Reduce heat to medium-low and continue to boil, stirring constantly until mixture thickens, 2 minutes. Remove from heat.
2. Beat eggs in a small mixing bowl, whisk in 1/3 of the hot milk mixture, then pour it back into the saucepan. Don't return to heat but continue to whisk until smooth and thick .Stir in lemon juice and peel.
3. Cover with waxed paper and refrigerate until cool. Stir in sour cream.
4. Fill 4 parfait glasses (or large wine glasses) with alternating layers of sliced strawberries and lemon cream.
5. Cover & chill until serving time (up to 8 hours).

Makes 4 servings.
Each serving of 1 parfait:
1 Fruit
1 Medium-fat meat

14g Carbohydrate, 6g Protein, 5g Fat, 123 cal
(14g available Carbohydrates)

Favorite Things

Heather's Dipping Sauce for Fruit

1 cup	Strawberry Yogurt, low fat
1/2 cup	'Light' sour cream
2 tbsp	'All fruit' strawberry spread or jam

Stir together and use as a dip for fresh fruit.

Exchanges for each serving of 1/8th recipe:

1 Vegetable

5g Carbohydrate, 2g Protein, 1g Fat, 23 cal

(5g available Carbohydrates)

Shannon's Late-For-School Breakfast

1/2	Banana, frozen, diced
1/2 cup	Soy milk
1/3 cup	Plain yogurt, low fat
1 tbsp	'Fat-reduced' peanut butter
2 tsp	Cocoa
1 tsp	Splenda®

Blend all ingredients in a food processor, blender, or with an electric wand.

Exchanges for each serving of 1 glass:

1/2 Starch	1 Low-fat milk
1/2 Fruit	1 Lean meat

29g Carbohydrate, 17g Protein, 7g Fat, 250 cal

(29g available Carbohydrates)

Jessica's Super Nachos for Two

12 large	Baked tortilla chips
1/2 cup	'Light' Cheddar cheese, grated
1/4 cup	Fat free refried beans
2 tbsp	Salsa

Arrange chips in a single layer on a large microwave-safe plate. Sprinkle with cheese. Top with beans and salsa. Microwave for 1 - 2 minutes.

Exchanges for each serving of 1/2 recipe:

1 1/2 Starch	1 Medium-fat meat

24g Carbohydrate, 12g Protein, 8g Fat, 125 cal

(24g available Carbohydrates)

Cream Cheese Frosting

8 oz	'Light' cream cheese
1/2 cup	Plain yogurt, low fat
1/3 cup	Splenda®
1/4 cup	Confectioners' sugar
1 tbsp	Orange juice
1 tsp	Orange peel
1 tsp	Vanilla extract

Stir cream cheese and yogurt together until smooth. Add remaining ingredients and beat until fluffy. Refrigerate until chilled.

Exchanges for each serving of 1/20th recipe:
1/4 Skim milk   1/2 Fat
3g Carbohydrate, 2g Protein, 2g Fat, 38 cal
(3g available Carbohydrates)

Willy's Cowboy Fajitas

4	8" Whole wheat tortillas
1	can (14oz) Pork & Beans
4	Turkey Weiners

Wrap tortillas in wax paper and warm in microwave for 1 minute, if desired. Heat beans in a small saucepan. Cook weiners in boiling water (or over a campfire) until hot. Spoon beans in the center of each tortilla. Top with a wiener. Roll up and serve.

Exchanges for each serving of 1 Fajita:
1 1 /2 Starch   1 1/2 Medium-fat meat
33g Carbohydrate, 14g Protein, 11g Fat, 198 cal
(33g available Carbohydrates)

Peachy Keen Slushy

1 cup	Peach yogurt, low fat
1 cup	Peach slices, canned

Mix in a food processor. Add 8 ice cubes, one at a time, blending until slushy.

Exchanges for each serving of 1 slushy:
1/2 Fruit   1/2 Skim milk
13g Carbohydrate, 4g Protein, 73kcal

Popcorn Munchios

8 cups	Popped popcorn
2 cups	Pretzels
2 cups	Crispix®
2 cups	Cheerios®
1 cup	Dry roasted peanuts
1 cup	Dried cranberries
1/4 cup	'Light' Italian dressing
1 tbsp	Honey mustard

1. Preheat oven to 300°F.
2. In a large bowl combine popcorn, pretzels, cereals, & peanuts.
3. In a small bowl stir together dressing and mustard. Pour over popcorn mixture and toss to coat evenly.
4. Spread on a baking sheet and bake for 25 to 30 mins, stirring once, until lightly toasted.

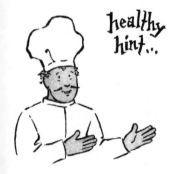

healthy hint...

Popcorn is a great low fat, low calorie snack food. Adding it to normally high fat 'Nuts and Bolts' recipes results in a great party snack! Experiment with your own additions.

Makes 8 servings.
Exchanges for each serving of 2 cups:
2 Starch   1 Fat
1/2 Medium-fat meat

31g Carbohydrate, 8g Protein, 10g Fat, 255 cal
(18g available Carbohydrates)

Index

Coq au vin	68	Full of beans salad	20
Corned beef hash frittata	53	Ginger orange chicken	62
Cowboy fajitas	158	Greek potatoes	27
Cream cheese frosting	158	Greek romaine salad	16
Crispy herbed sole	84	Greek tomato bake	23
Crunchy parmesan chicken	67	Grilled banana sundae	143
Curried chicken salad	21	Grilled chicken caesar salad	22
Deep dish tuna pie	92	Grilled halibut burgers	81
Dipping sauce for fruit	157	Hearty carrot muffins	36
Double chocolate cupcakes	151	Ham & pineapple kabobs	106
Dude ranch dip	2	Hot Chinese chicken salad	70
Easy apple crisp	147	Hot German potato salad	26
Eggs		Hot tamale pie	113

Eggs
- Breakfast in a bun — 48
- Cheese & veggie strata — 55
- Corned beef hash frittata — 53
- Eggs Benny — 50
- Farmer's casserole — 52
- Huevos rancheros — 51
- No crust quiche — 54
- Overnight egg scramble — 49

Eggs Benny — 50
Farmer's Casserole — 52
Fast & healthy stir-fry — 100

Fish & Seafood
- Baked fish picante — 87
- Cod crumble — 89
- Crispy herbed sole — 84
- Deep dish tuna pie — 92
- Fish & chips — 88
- Fresh salsa snapper — 86
- Grilled halibut burgers — 81
- Layered tuna salad — 17
- Lemon shrimp & scallop kabobs — 80
- Marinated shrimp — 12
- Mexi cod with pasta shells — 90
- Pepper sole Veronique — 85
- Salmon gremolata — 82
- Salmon & lemony mayo — 83
- Salmon & rice casserole — 93
- Salmon strudel — 94
- Stuffed mushroom caps — 5
- Tuna tetrazzini — 91

Fish & chips — 88
Fresh salsa snapper — 86
Fruit & nut drops — 130
Fruit slushy — 158
Fruity Clafouti — 60

Full of beans salad — 20
Ginger orange chicken — 62
Greek potatoes — 27
Greek romaine salad — 16
Greek tomato bake — 23
Grilled banana sundae — 143
Grilled chicken caesar salad — 22
Grilled halibut burgers — 81
Hearty carrot muffins — 36
Ham & pineapple kabobs — 106
Hot Chinese chicken salad — 70
Hot German potato salad — 26
Hot tamale pie — 113
Huevos rancheros — 51
Idaho chili stew — 115
Jamaiican jerk chicken — 65
Late-for-school breakfast — 157
Layered Mexican dip — 14
Layered tuna salad — 17
Lazy day peach pie — 152
Lemon cookies — 129
Lemon shrimp & scallop kabobs — 80
Marbled cheesecake squares — 138
Marinated shrimp — 12
Maui meatball kabobs — 76
Mexi cod with pasta shells — 90
Mexican chicken spirals — 4
Monte Cristo sandwiches — 59

Muffins & Breads
- Apple walnut muffins — 39
- Banana bran nut loaf — 46
- Blueberry-raspberry muffins — 35
- Bran muffins — 34
- Cheesy corn muffins — 38
- Cinnamon rolls — 45
- Hearty carrot muffins — 36
- Pepper & herb foccacia — 44
- Perfect popovers — 41
- Pumpkin chocolate chip muffins — 37
- Red pepper corn bread — 43
- Tender flaky biscuits — 42
- Zucchini & dill muffins — 40

Mushroom gravy — 99
Mushroom pizza bread — 10
Mushroom & spinach lasagna — 121
New potato salad — 19
New wave waldorf salad — 18
No crust quiche — 54

First Choice Cookbook

Order Form

Order **FIRST CHOICE COOKBOOK** at $13.95(U.S.) per book
plus $4.00 (total order) for shipping and handling.

Order **KIDS CHOICE COOKBOOK** at $11.95(U.S.) per book
plus $4.00 (total order) for shipping and handling
(U.S. and international orders payable in U.S. funds.)

Number of books

First Choice Cookbook _____   x **$13.95** = _____

Kids Choice Cookbook _____   x **$11.95** = _____

Postage & Handling: $4.00 (total order)   _____

Total: _____

Name: _____

Street: _____

City: _____   State: _____

Country: _____   Zip: _____

Make cheque or money order payable to:
Picnics Publishing
Box 2461 Sechelt
B.C., Canada   V0N 3A0

For large volume orders fax 604-885-4375